Updated & Revised Fifth Edition

82 SUBJECTS COVERED!

DR. TEMPLE GRANDIN

THE WAY I SEE IT

A Personal Look at Autism

Foreword by Tony Attwood, PhD

The Way I See It:
A Personal Look at Autism

All marketing and publishing rights guaranteed to and reserved by:

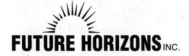

FUTURE HORIZONS INC.

800-489-0727 (toll free)
817-277-0727 (local)
817-277-2270 (fax)
E-mail: *info@fhautism.com*
www.fhautism.com
© 2020 Temple Grandin
Cover and interior design, John Yacio III
All rights reserved.
Printed in Canada.

Cover and interior photos © Rosalie Winard: Cow photo in chapter title collage, author bio, and central photos on titles for chapters 2, 3, 8, and 9.

Chapter 4 title image © Angus Bremner.

ISBN: 9781949177312

Contents

Foreword ....*vii*

Foreword to the Second Edition ....*ix*

Foreword to the First Edition ....*xiii*

For Readers New to Autism..*xxi*

Introduction ....*xxv*

Chapter 1: The Importance of Early Education 1

The Importance of Early Educational Intervention 3

Do Not Get Trapped by Labels...9

Economical Quality Programs for Young Children with ASD 18

Different Types of Thinking in Autism..21

Higher Expectations Yield Results 28

Teaching Turn Taking...32

What School Is Best for My Child with ASD?......................................34

Chapter 2: Teaching & Education 37

Finding a Child's Area of Strength..46

Teaching How to Generalize 49

The Importance of Developing Talent 52

Teaching People on the Autism Spectrum to Be More Flexible 54

Teaching Concepts to Children with Autism 56

Bottom-Up Thinking and Learning Rules...58

Laying the Foundation for Reading Comprehension 63

Motivating Students 67

Getting Kids Turned On to Reading..71

Too Much Video Gaming and Screen Time has a Bad Effect on Child Development...74

Therapy Animals and Autism 82

The Importance of Choices 91

The Importance of Practical Problem-Solving Skills...........................94

Learning to Do Assignments That Other People Appreciate 97

Learning Never Stops..100

Chapter 3: Sensory Issues 103

Sensory Problems Are Variable 107

Visual Processing Problems in Autism..115

Auditory Processing Problems and Sound Over Sensitivity in Autism
....120

Incorporating Sensory Methods into Your Autism Program...............126

The Effect of Sensory and Perceptual Difficulties on Learning Patterns
....131

Environmental Enrichment Therapy for Autism 136

Chapter 4: Understanding Nonverbal Autism..................139

A Social Teenager Trapped Inside..153

You Asked Me! 156

Why Do Kids with Autism Stim? 159

Tito Lives in a World of Sensory Scrambling 162

Understanding the Mind of a Nonverbal Person with Autism............165

Solving Behavior Problems in Nonverbal Individuals with Autism 169

Whole-Task Teaching for Individuals with Severe Autism 174

Chapter 5: Behavior Issues...177

Disability versus Just Bad Behaviors..182

My Experience with Teasing and Bullying 186

Rudeness is Inexcusable..190

The Need to Be Perfect..193

Contents

Autism & Religion: Teach Goodness..197

Chapter 6: Social Functioning...*201*

Insights into Autistic Social Problems..211

Learning Social Rules 213

Emotional Differences Among Individuals with Autism or Asperger's

....216

Healthy Self-Esteem..219

Four Cornerstones of Social Awareness 222

Questions about Connecticut Shooter Adam Lanza, Asperger's Syndrome, and SPD...225

Chapter 7: Medications & Biomedical Issues....................*229*

Alternative Versus Conventional Medicine 248

Autism Medical Update...255

Hidden Medical Problems Can Cause Behavior Problems....................260

Evaluating Treatments 264

Medication Usage: Risk versus Benefit Decisions..............................268

My Treatment for Ringingin the Ears...279

Chapter 8: Cognition & Brain Research *283*

Chapter 9: Adult Issues & Employment *295*

Improving Time Management and Organizational Skills....................306

Employment Advice: Tips for Getting and Holding a Job 309

Teens with ASD Must Learn Both Social and Work Skills to Keep Jobs

....314

Happy People on the Autism Spectrum Have Satisfying Jobs or

Hobbies..318

Inside or Outside? The Autism/Asperger's Culture..............................321

Portfolios Can Open Job and College Opportunities 325

Going to College: Tips for People with Autism & Asperger's 328

Finding Mentors and Appropriate Colleges...................................... 333

Reasonable Accommodation for Individuals on the Autism Spectrum
....336

Get Out and Experience Life! 340

Can My Adolescent Drive a Car?.. 343

Innovative Thinking Paves the Way for AS Career Success.............. 347

Try on Careers 350

The Link Between Autism Genetics and Genius 354

My Sense of Self-Identity 359

Tony & Temple: Face to Face *363*

Bibliography...*375*

About the Author *381*

Foreword

I have known Temple for over twenty-five years and have always admired her understanding of autism, which is based not only on her personal experiences but also her extensive knowledge of the research literature. Temple has an amazing ability to entrance audiences and readers with her insights and explanations. She is a very forthright person, and I can "hear" her voice on every page.

Temple's revised *The Way I See It* is a compilation of articles from the *Autism Asperger's Digest* over twenty years. It is interesting that her insightful conceptualization of autism over two decades has continued to be confirmed by independent research and clinical experience.

This revision covers a wide range of topics across the entire autism spectrum, from self-injurious behavior and communication difficulties in severe autism to issues regarding college and employment for those who are able to be self-sufficient and achieve a successful career. Temple provides wise advice on contemporary issues such as the changing diagnostic criteria, the recommended amount of daily screen time, and the advantages of therapy animals. Temple also provides relevant academic references and her personally recommended resources for each article and chapter. In reading this book, parents, those who have autism, professionals, and especially teachers will all achieve a greater appreciation of the qualities and challenges associated with autism.

I know that I will be taking quotes and metaphors from *The Way I See It* to illustrate specific points in my clinical work and presentations, and I will be advising colleagues that their expertise will be greatly enhanced by reading Temple's explanations and recommendations. I will also advise clients to read her new book to achieve a greater degree of self-understanding by absorbing her wisdom and positive approach to autism. In reading *The Way I See It*, you too will see autism the way it is.

PROFESSOR TONY ATTWOOD

Foreword to the Second Edition

by Emily Gerson Saines

Producer of the HBO *Temple Grandin* Movie

and Mother of a Child with Autism

Autism entered my life prior to my son Dashiell's second birthday. We, like so many parents, told our pediatricians of what are now known to be the classic signs of autism. Our son lost his language, began spinning, flapping his hands, having tantrums, and withdrew into his own world, a world into which we were not invited. For almost a year, we went to his pediatrician's office to discuss these behaviors, only to be told there was nothing to worry about; he was simply experiencing his terrible twos. However, his behaviors escalated, and we witnessed him becoming a danger to himself and others. We called the pediatrician and said, "This is not just the terrible twos. Something is wrong—something is horribly wrong." We insisted that my son be tested, and within a few short hours of arriving at the hospital, we were told that our son was diagnosed with Pervasive Developmental Disorder (PDD). For many of us, being given a diagnosis of PDD is a gentle way of saying, "Your child, your beautiful baby with ten fingers and ten toes, has autism. He may never be able to read, write, talk, or hold down a job. He may never live alone, have friends, be welcomed into a community, marry, or have a family of his own."

The next several months were equally brutal. Our school district had an early intervention pre-kindergarten program. They assured us that the teacher was well trained and that the school was well equipped to handle him. We enrolled him, and on the first day of school, they lost him—physically lost him. Upon closer examination, it turned out this so-called "well-trained" teacher had never taught a child with autism—ever. Being two well-educated parents, we were confident that we could do a better job on our own. We set up a home-based program to be run by one of the most highly regarded behavioral therapists at the time. Unfortunately our timing was off, as our highly regarded behavioral therapist was in the midst of a nervous breakdown and as a result, her "therapy" methods more so resembled child abuse than teaching. We couldn't have felt more lost, more alone, and more inadequate when one day, a package from my mother arrived in the mail. It was a book called *Thinking in Pictures* by Temple Grandin. The following day, an envelope from my grandmother arrived, and in it a *New Yorker* article written by Oliver Sacks about none other than Temple Grandin.

Temple's story is remarkable. She is a gifted animal scientist, the most successful designer of humane livestock handling facilities in the United States, and she has autism. She began life nonverbal and with a variety of inappropriate behaviors. In spite of her autism, today she can read, she can write, she can talk (boy can she talk), she lives on her own, she can hold down a job (in fact she has many of them), she is a consultant for a number of Fortune 500 companies, she is a best-selling author, she is a lecturer (on livestock and autism), she is a professor of Animal Science at Colorado State University, and perhaps most importantly, she is a friend—a dear friend. She is fiercely loyal, always available, and willing to take action. Once upon a time, all of this seemed like a pipedream even for Temple, but with the support and encouragement of her mother, Eustacia Cutler, and other mentors in her life, Temple went from being a nonverbal four-year-old to being all she is today. For parents of children with autism, Temple Grandin is our hero. She has given us a window into our children's minds and a reclaimed dream for a future filled with possibilities.

Thirteen years ago, I realized that Temple's story needed to be shared with a wider audience. As I transitioned from being an agent at the

William Morris Agency into owning my own management company, I realized it was possible for me to lead that charge and produce a film about her extraordinary life. I called Temple, reached out to HBO, and we were on our way. It took us ten years to get it right, but I couldn't be more proud of our film, *Temple Grandin*, which celebrates the life of someone I respect and admire so much. Whether I was sharing a meal with her in New York, reviewing dailies with her in my hotel room in Austin, sitting beside her at the Golden Globes, being hugged by her on stage at the Emmys, or listening to her encourage the Chairman of Time Warner to examine the McDonald's distribution system, my days with Temple have been amongst the best and most interesting of my life.

After settling back into my normal life, I picked up a copy of Temple's book *The Way I See It.* Just when I thought I had learned everything Temple could teach me, I was astonished to learn there was more—a lot more. Often parents of children with autism are encouraged to adhere to a routine with their child.

Temple devotes an entire chapter to encouraging flexibility in a routine and provides examples on how to accomplish that. She identifies strategies for encouraging interests that can later become vocations, as children with autism become adults with autism. Additionally, Temple reminds us that learning is a continuum. Human beings have the ability to learn well into their senior years, and the exposure to new things is essential in expanding a person's mind, even, and perhaps especially, if they have autism. This book is insightful, helpful, and hopeful—just like the woman who wrote it! It is a "how-to" guide that I am confident will leave any reader feeling both informed and inspired.

EMILY GERSON SAINES

February 2011

Foreword to the First Edition

by Dr. Ruth Sullivan

Director of the First National Autism Society

Who better than Temple Grandin to give us a personal look at autism and Asperger's?

For over thirty of her nearly sixty years' experience on the autism spectrum, Temple has dedicated much of her time, energy, considerable intellect, and talents to learning about her condition and translating it for the rest of us. This book puts together under one cover her highly insightful, informed, articulate, and most of all, practical, ideas and instructions for dealing with the wide range of behaviors, learning styles, and physical health issues found in autism and Asperger's Syndrome.

At the time Temple came on the autism scene, few people had heard of autism, and even fewer had ever heard of someone with autism who could communicate well enough to tell us how it felt, from the inside. I was a member of a small group of parents of children with autism, nationwide, who in November 1965, at the invitation of Dr. Bernard Rimland, met to form a national organization, the National Society for Autistic Children (NSAC), now called the Autism Society of America (ASA). Our goal was to seek a better understanding of this mysterious condition that so severely affected our children, and to seek treatment, as well as cause and cure. There was almost nothing in the literature. Dr. Rimland's book, *Infantile Autism: The Syndrome and Its Implications for a Neural Theory of Behavior* (published in 1964) was among the very first on the subject. None of us knew an adult with autism.

I first met Temple in the mid-1980s at the St. Louis Airport, when making a connection to Chicago for the annual NSAC conference. In the small waiting area there were about 25 other conference goers from across the nation, also waiting for that flight. Most of us knew each other, and the talk was mostly about autism.

Standing on the periphery of the group was a tall young woman who was obviously interested in the discussions. She seemed shy and pleasant, but mostly she just listened. Once in Chicago, she and I got on the conference bus and sat together as we traveled to our hotel. I learned her name was Temple Grandin, and this was her first autism conference. I was impressed at how much she knew about the condition. It wasn't until later in the week that I realized she was someone with autism. I had heard of a woman who had that diagnosis, who was high-functioning, but had not connected the two. I approached her and asked if she'd be willing to speak at the next year's NSAC conference program. She agreed.

Back then, NSAC conferences were the only national meetings focused solely on autism. Each year there was one entire session set aside just for information exchange. It was held in a large room of ten-person round tables, each designated for a special subject, with a discussion leader. That next year I was the discussion leader for a table labeled "Adults with Autism," and that's where Temple first addressed an NSAC audience. The ten chairs were filled immediately, and people were standing at least three deep. The room became noisy, and with so many wanting to hear every word Temple said, I asked for a room just for us. More people followed as we were led to a small auditorium.

Temple and I stood on the slightly elevated stage. The audience couldn't get enough of her. Here, for the first time, was someone who could tell us from her own experience what it was like to be extremely sound sensitive ("like being tied to the rail and the train's coming"). On the topic of wearing certain kinds of underwear, she described her profound skin sensitivity, and how she could not verbally articulate how painful it was. On relationships, she talked about how hard it was to communicate what she felt, and about her difficulty in understanding others. She was asked many questions: "Why does my son do so much spinning?" "What can I do about toilet training?" "Why does he hold his hands to his ears?" "Why doesn't he look at me?" She spoke from her own experience, and her insight was impressive. There were tears in more than one set of eyes that day.

After the hour-long session ended, many stayed around to talk to Temple. She seemed surprised but pleased with the attention—even adulation. Later, when I asked, she said she had been a little nervous. Over the years, I've often thought about that scene, and marveled at how remarkable an event it was for her, and all of us.

Not long afterwards, in 1986, her first book was published, *Emergence: Labeled Autistic*. The rest is history, as they say. Ten years later came her highly acclaimed work, *Thinking in Pictures*, with other autism books to follow. Temple simultaneously became well known for her work and writings in her chosen professional field of animal behavior. She earned a Ph.D. in that discipline, from the University of Colorado. Her 2006 release, *Animals in Translation*, became a *New York Times* Bestseller.

Temple quickly became a much sought-after speaker in the autism community. She wrote articles for the popular press as well as peer reviewed professional journals. Always generous to projects related to parents and their children, she wrote for parent organization newsletters, and traveled around the U.S. and the world to speak at autism conferences. Probably no one with autism has appeared in the world media more than Temple, nor had a bigger impact on our global understanding of autism and Asperger's Syndrome and the people diagnosed on the spectrum.

Yet, the Temple Grandin of today is not the same woman I met nearly twenty-five years ago. It has been a remarkable privilege to witness

Temple's growth in social skills and awareness throughout the time I have known her. She is one of the hardest workers I have ever known. In my opinion, it is mainly that trait that has helped her become the successful, engaging adult she is now, despite severe difficulties along the way. She is knowledgeable. She is willing to help parents as well as others with autism. She is insightful. And she is courageous—a fitting word to explain her heartfelt, strong (and sometimes unwanted) advice to her adult peers with autism or Asperger's on the importance of being polite, dressing appropriately, accepting responsibility for their actions and following rules of civility if they want to get and keep a job or have friends.

And not least, she is funny. Though generally her presentations are straightforward, in recent years she has become quite good at humor. Her audiences love it.

In addition, and to her credit, she has learned to be generous in recognizing those who have helped her along the way, namely her mother, Eustacia Cutler, whose book, *A Thorn in My Pocket*, tells the family story. Others are teachers and colleagues who saw her potential and bravely went beyond current practice to help her develop some of her strengths. For many individuals with autism, it is difficult-to-impossible to understand and develop "theory of mind," that intangible mental process by which most of us intuitively notice and "read" the nuances of social situations: how others are feeling, what they may be thinking, and the meaning behind their nonverbal actions. Temple's persistence in learning this, and her strong analytical skills while doing so, have helped significantly in improving her social thinking and social sense.

Temple continues to wrap her energies around autism and the people it touches. Her talent is a gift to all of us—not just those of us in the autism community, but the world at large. The book you are holding in your hand is the result of her keen detective-like analysis of human beings, her extensive personal thought, and the wisdom gained only through the personal experiences that make up Temple Grandin. It serves as an excellent summary of what one human being has contributed to one of the most disabling and puzzling conditions known to mankind. Temple takes time to listen—without pre-conceived ideas or judgment—to parents and the professionals who work with and for individuals with autism on the entire spectrum, from severe autism to high-level Asperger's. She seeks solutions, from teaching strategies to the larger lifespan issues that can present challenges of immense proportions, even for neurotypicals. The suggestions she offers in this book are imaginative, well thought out, practical, and useful. She talks directly to the reader, with honesty and understanding. She knows what autism is like, and her recommendations make sense.

Every library, large or small, needs this book on its shelves. Every school, large or small, with the responsibility of educating children with autism or Asperger's, needs the guidance this book offers. Every teacher within those schools will benefit from reading it and applying the strategies Temple so clearly illuminates. Last, and certainly not least, every parent will find within these pages golden nuggets of advice, encouragement, and hope to fuel their day-to-day journey through their child's autism.

As I've heard Temple often remark in the twenty-something years I have known her, about the way she views autism and her life: "I didn't become social overnight. There wasn't a point when some magic switch turned on in my brain and the social stuff made sense after that. I'm the person I am today because of all the experiences I've had, and the opportunities those experiences offered me to learn, little by little. It wasn't easy; sometimes it was really difficult. I've made a lot of mistakes, but I just kept going until I got it right. And, I'm still learning today!

That's what I want other people on the spectrum to learn: You just can't give up. You have to keep trying." The wisdom she offers through this book and its personal reflections on autism will, I'm sure, ring true for many more decades to come.

RUTH CHRIST SULLIVAN, PH.D.

May 2008

Ruth Christ Sullivan, Ph.D. was the first elected president of the Autism Society of America (formerly NSAC), founded in 1965 by the late Dr. Bernard Rimland. In 1979 she founded and was Executive Director of Autism Services Center (ASC), in Huntington, WV until her retirement in 2007, at age 83. ASC is a nonprofit, licensed behavioral health care agency that serves all developmental disabilities but specializes in comprehensive, autism-specific services, in community-based settings including clients' homes. ASC serves approximately 270 clients, with a staff of 350. Dr. Sullivan was one of the chief autism lobbyists for Public Law 94-142 (now known as the Individuals with Disabilities Education Act, IDEA), as well as the Developmental Disabilities Act. She was the main force behind the founding of the West Virginia Autism Training Center at Marshall University, in Huntington, WV, in 1983.

Dr. Sullivan assisted in the production of the 1988 movie, *Rain Man*, serving as a consultant on autism behavior. Dustin Hoffman, who won an Oscar for his starring role as Raymond Babbett, worked directly with Dr. Sullivan and her son, Joseph (born in 1960), who has autism, in practicing for his role. The premiere of *Rain Man* was held in Huntington with Dustin Hoffman and Barry Levinson, the producer, present. It was a benefit event for Autism Services Center.

Though Dr. Sullivan has lived in Huntington, WV for forty years, she is still close to her large, south Louisiana Cajun family in Lake Charles.

For Readers New to Autism

Autism is a developmental disorder, typically diagnosed during early childhood. It is neurological in nature, affecting the brain in four major areas of functioning: language/communication, social skills, sensory systems, and behavior. Current research suggests there may be different subsets of the disorder arising from genetics, environmental insults, or a combination of both. Do not panic if your child is diagnosed with autism. When I was 2½ years old, I had no speech, constant tantrums, and repetitive behavior. Intensive early speech therapy and turn-taking games were effective. Today I am a university professor of animal science at Colorado State University. When kids are under five years of age, it is difficult to predict how they will develop. Some socially awkward children receive an autism diagnosis in either high school or elementary school because they have no friends. These children can benefit greatly from programs that teach social skills. Some of these kids are brilliant and can have a good career in computer science, art, engineering, or a highly skilled trade. During my career designing livestock equipment for many major corporations, I worked with many skilled people who were probably undiagnosed individuals with autism, ADHD, or dyslexia.

Every person with autism is unique, with a different profile of strengths and challenges. No two individuals manifest the same characteristics in the same degree of severity. It is a "spectrum" disorder, and the various individual diagnoses are collectively referred to as autism spectrum disorder (ASD). Individuals on the spectrum range from those who remain nonverbal with severe challenges that can include self-injurious behaviors and intellectual disability to individuals on the fully verbal end of the spectrum (known as Asperger's syndrome under old guidelines), who are extremely intelligent with good expressive verbal language yet markedly impaired social skills and weak perspective-taking abilities. The autism spectrum is very broad, ranging from socially awkward brilliant workers in Silicon Valley to individuals who will always have to live in a supervised living situation. Some kids on the high end of the autism spectrum are gifted in art, music, or mathematics. In 2013, changes were made in diagnostic criteria in the DSM (Diagnostic and Statistical Manual of Mental Disorders), the diagnostic "bible" of the U.S. medical community, which eliminated Asperger's syndrome. The various autism labels are now merged into one designation, "autism spectrum disorders." An autism diagnosis is not precise. Over the years, committees of doctors have kept changing the diagnostic criteria. A draft of the new ICD-11 international autism diagnostic guidelines has been published. It may provide a clearer guidance to both parents and professionals.

The rate of autism is now 1 in every 59 births (Centers for Disease Control, 2019) and continues to escalate at alarming rates. Every 21 minutes, a child is diagnosed on the spectrum. It is four times more common in boys than girls and is consistently prevalent around the globe within different racial, social, and ethnic communities. According to the Autism Society of America, the lifetime cost of caring for a single child with severe autism ranges from $3.5 to $5 million.

Autism is a different way of thinking and learning. People with autism are people first. Autism is only one part of who they are. ASD is no longer viewed as strictly a behavioral disorder, but one that affects the whole person on various fronts: biomedical, cognitive, social, and sensory. With individualized and appropriate intervention, children with ASD can become more functional and learn to adapt to the world around them.

Great strides are being made in our understanding of autism spectrum disorders and how best to help these individuals. Children are now being diagnosed as early as 12 to 15 months old and many who receive intensive early intervention are able to enter elementary school in class with their typical peers, needing minor supports and services. No matter the age of diagnosis, children and adults with ASD are constant learners and significant improvements in their functioning can be made at any age with the appropriate types and intensity of services.

Too many parents coddle and overprotect their children. I am seeing teenagers who are fully verbal and doing well academically not learning life skills such as shopping, bank account or keeping and holding a job. My mother made sure I learned all these things when I was a teenager and a young adult. She always gave me choices of new things to try, but I was not allowed to be a recluse in my room all day. However, I had some scheduled time to be alone to calm down. Today I talk to many grandparents who discover that they are on the autism spectrum when their grandchildren are diagnosed. These grandparents learned life skills when they were young and many of them had excellent careers.

Introduction

This fifth edition of this book is a compilation of articles I have written for the *Autism Asperger's Digest* magazine from the year 2000 to the present. The articles have been grouped into different categories, addressing subjects from early educational interventions, to sensory sensitivity problems, to brain research and careers. At the beginning of each section I have added a new, updated introduction, which includes additional thoughts on the subject matter. Articles that required updating were updated.

The articles combine both my personal experiences with autism and practical information that parents, teachers, and individuals on the autism spectrum can put to immediate use. The autism spectrum is very broad, ranging from individuals who remain nonverbal to a mild Asperger's individual who is a brilliant scientist or computer engineer. This book contains information that can be applied across the entire autism spectrum.

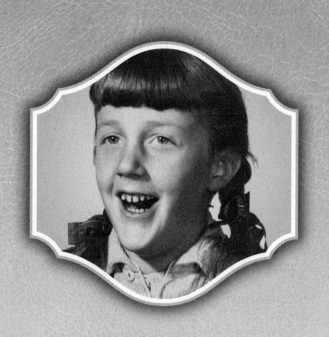

CHAPTER 1

The Importance of Early Education

The best thing a parent of a newly diagnosed child can do is to watch their child, without preconceived notions and judgments, and learn how the child functions, acts, and reacts to his or her world.

The Importance of Early Educational Intervention

B oth research and practical experience show that an intensive early education program in which a young child receives a minimum of twenty hours a week of instruction from a skilled teacher greatly improves prognosis. The brain of the young child is still growing and evolving. At this age, the neural pathways are highly malleable, and intensive instruction can reprogram "faulty wiring" that prevents the child from learning. Plus, behaviors in a young child have not yet become ingrained. It will take less practice to change an inappropriate behavior at age two to three than it will to change the same behavior at age seven to eight. By then, the child has had many years of doing things his way and change comes about more slowly.

For early childhood programs, ABA (applied behavioral analysis) programs using discrete trial training have the best scientific documentation backing up their use. But other programs, such as the Denver early start program, have been validated in a randomized trial. Additional evidence-based programs are pivotal response, speech therapy, and occupational therapy. The autism spectrum is vast and diversified. Children have different ways of thinking and processing information, and it is important that an intervention method be aligned with the child's learning profile and personality. Detailed descriptions of different types of early intervention programs can be found online.

A book I recommend is Early Intervention and Autism: Real Life Questions, Real Life Answers by Dr. James Ball (2012) from Future Horizons,

Inc. While this book is written for parents of newly diagnosed children, more than three-quarters of the information on interventions, effective teaching strategies, program planning, and behavior management is valuable for parents of children of all ages.

My Early Intervention Program

I had a wonderful effective early education program that started at age two and a half. By then, I had all the classic symptoms of autism including no speech, no eye contact, tantrums, and constant repetitive behavior. In 1949 when I was two-and-a-half years old, the doctors knew nothing about autism, but my mother would not accept that nothing could be done to help me. She was determined, and knew that letting me continue without treatment would be the worst thing she could do. She obtained advice from a wise neurologist who referred her to a speech therapist to work with me. She was just as good as the autism specialists today.

My talented speech therapist worked with me for three hours a week doing ABA-type training (breaking skills down into small components, teaching each component separately using repetitive drills that gave me lots of practice) and she carefully enunciated hard consonant sounds so I could hear them. At the speech therapy school, I also attended a highly structured nursery school class with five or six other children who were not autistic. Several of the children had Down syndrome. These classes lasted about eight hours a week.

My nanny was another critical part of my early therapy. She spent 20 hours a week keeping me engaged. For instance, playing repeated turn-taking games with my sister and me. She was instrumental in introducing early social skills lessons, even though at that time, they weren't referred to as such in a formal manner. Within the realm of play, she kept me engaged and set up activities so that most involved turn-taking and lessons about being with others. In the winter, we went outdoors to play in the snow. She brought one sled and my sister and I had to take turns sledding down the hill. In the summer, we took turns on the swing. We were also taught to sit at the table and have good table manners. Teaching and learning opportunities were woven into everyday life.

When I turned five, we played lots of board games such as Parcheesi and Chinese checkers. My interest in art and making things was actively encouraged and I did many art projects. For most of the day, I was forced to keep my brain tuned into the world. However, my mother realized that my behaviors served a purpose and that changing those behaviors didn't happen overnight. I was given one hour after lunch where I could revert back to repetitive autistic behaviors without consequence. During this hour, I had to stay in my room. I sometimes spent the entire time spinning a decorative brass plate that covered a bolt that held my bed frame together. I would spin it at different speeds and was fascinated at how different speeds affected the number of times the brass plate spun.

The best thing a parent of a newly diagnosed child can do is to watch their child without preconceived notions and judgements and learn how the child functions, acts, and reacts to his or her world. That information will be invaluable in finding an intervention method that will be a good match to the child's learning style and needs. The worst thing parents can do with a child between the ages of two to five is nothing. It doesn't matter if the child is formally diagnosed with autism spectrum disorder (ASD) or has been labeled something less defined, such as global developmental delay. It doesn't matter if the child is not yet diagnosed if there are signs that the child may be on the spectrum: speech is severely delayed, the child's behaviors are odd and repetitive, the child doesn't engage with people or his/her environment, etc. The child must not be allowed to sit around stimming all day or, conversely, tuning out the world around him/her. Parents, hear this: doing nothing is the worst thing you can do. If you have a three-year-old with no speech who is showing signs of autistic behavior, you need to start working with your child now. If signs are appearing in a child younger than three, even better. Do not wait six more months or a year even if your pediatrician is suggesting you take the "wait and see" approach or is plying you with advice such as "boys develop later than girls" or "not all children start to speak at the same time." My advice to act now is doubly emphasized if your child's language started developing late or his/her language and/or behavior is regressing.

Parents can find themselves on long waiting lists for both diagnosis and early intervention services. In some cases, the child will age out of the state's early intervention system (birth to three) before his name gets to the top of the list! There is much parents can do to begin working with the child before formal professional intervention begins. Play turn-taking games and encourage eye contact. Grandmothers who have lots of experience with children can be very effective. If you are unable to obtain professional services for your young child, you need to start working with your child immediately.

This book and Raun Kaufman's book, Autism Breakthrough, will be useful guides on how to work with young kids. The best part of Kaufman's book are the teaching guidelines that grandmothers and other untrained people can easily use. Ignore his opinions about other treatments. Do not allow young children under five to zone out with tablets, phones, or other electronic devices. In young children, solitary screen time must be limited to one hour a day. For children under five, all other activities with electronic devices should be interactive activities done with a parent or teacher.

The intense interest in the electronic device can be used to motivate interest in doing a game where turns are taken with another person. During this game, the phone should be physically passed back and forth during turn taking. Too many kids are tuning out the world with electronics. In older children, video game playing should be limited to one hour a day. Excessive video gaming and screen use is a major problem in individuals with autism.

Engagement with the child at this point in time is just as effective as is instruction. While you may not yet be knowledgeable about various autism intervention models, you are smart enough and motivated enough to engage your child for 20 plus hours a week. Don't wait! Act now!

References and Additional Reading

Adele, D. (2017) The impact of delay of early intensive behavioral intervention on educational outcomes for a cohort of medicaid-enrolled children with autism, *Dissertation*, University of Minnesota.

Ball, J. (2012) *Early Intervention and Autism: Real Life Questions, Real Life Answers*, Future Horizons, Inc., Arlington, TX.

Children's Hospital of Philadelphia (2017) Evidence-based treatment options for Autism, www.chop.edu/news/evidence-based-treatment-options-autism (Accessed June 22, 2019).

Dawson, G. et al. (2010) Randomized controlled trial of an intervention for toddlers with autism: The Early Start Mode, *Pediatrics* 125:e17-e23.

Grandin, T. (1996) *Emergence: Labeled Autistic*, Warner, Books, New York NY.

Gengoux, G.W. et al. (2019) A pivotal response treatment package for children with autism spectrum disorder, *Pediatrics*, Sept:144(3) doi:10.1542/peds.2019-0178

Kaufman, R.K. (2015) *Autism Breakthrough*, St. Martin's Griffin.

Koegel, L. and Lazebnik, C. (2014) *Overcoming Autism: Finding Strategies and Hope That Can Transport a Child's Life*, Penguin Group, New York, NY.

Le, J. and Ventola, P. (2017) Pivotal response treatment for autism spectrum disorder: *Current Perspectives in Neuropsychiatric Disorders Treatment*, 13:1613-1626.

Do Not Get Trapped by Labels

An autism diagnosis is not precise, like a diagnosis for a disease. I can get a lab test for cancer or tuberculosis that is very definitive; this is not true for autism. In the U.S., a diagnosis for autism is a behavioral profile based on a manual published by the American Psychiatric Association called the DSM (Diagnostic and Statistical Manual of Mental Disorders). The behavioral profiles in this manual are based on a combination of scientific studies and the opinion of a panel of expert doctors who debated in a conference room. A draft of the new ICD-11 (International Classification of Diseases) guidelines was published in 2019. It will be outlined in this chapter. Since the ICD is used in many countries around the world for all types of diseases, it is designed to be easily used by primary care doctors.

When Richard Panek and I worked on our book titled *The Autistic Brain* (2013), we reviewed the entire history of the DSM. Since the 1950s and 1960s, the diagnostic criteria for autism has changed dramatically. When all the changes made during the last 60 years are looked at side-by-side, it is rather shocking.

In 1980, a child had to have both speech delay and autistic behaviors to be diagnosed with autism. In 1994, Asperger's syndrome was added, in which the child is socially awkward with no speech delay. In the 2013 DSM-5 (American Psychiatric Association), Asperger's syndrome (AS) and PDD-NOS (pervasive developmental disorder—not otherwise specified) were removed. These labels are now all merged into a broad autism spectrum disorder (ASD). There is no longer any requirement for speech delay. Taking out speech delay makes the DSM-5 more vague than the old DSM-IV. Some scientists do not consider language delay as a core symptom of autism because language delays and speech abnormalities are so variable.

For a person to be labeled with ASD, the DSM-5 requires that symptoms must be present in early childhood, but the age of onset is no longer defined. The DSM-5 whittles symptoms down to social and behavioral. The main emphasis is on social abnormalities inherent in the disorder: deficits in social interaction, reciprocal communication, and developing and keeping relationships with friends. In addition, the child must have two out of four of the following: repetitive behavior, adherence to routines, fixated interests, or sensory problems. Studies have shown that 91 percent of individuals with an Asperger's or PDD-NOS diagnosis will still quality for an ASD diagnosis in the DSM-5. The DSM-5 also created a new social communication diagnosis, which consists of the social problems of ASD without the repetitive behavior, fixated interests, or sensory problems. To state that this is not autism does not make sense, because social deficits are a core autism symptom. Since there is no funding for social communication disorder, very few children have received this diagnosis.

Autism is a Huge Spectrum

One of the big problems with autism (ASD) diagnosis is that it has now changed to a broad spectrum with a wide-ranging degree of abilities. When children are really little (age two to five), most experts agree that many early educational treatments greatly improve prognosis. When I was three, I had no speech and all the typical autistic symptoms. ABA-type (applied behavior analysis) speech therapy and turn-taking games made it possible for me to be enrolled in a regular kindergarten at age five.

Rebecca Grzadzinski, Marisela Huerta, and Catherine Lord (2013) stated, "In terms of cognitive functioning, individuals with ASD display a wide range of abilities from severe intellectual disability (ID) to superior intelligence."

Individuals with ASD range from computer scientists at Silicon Valley to individuals who will never live independently. They may not be able to participate in activities such as shopping trips or a sports event. When such a broad range of abilities is lumped together, it is difficult for special education teachers to shift gears between the different levels of abilities. Too often a child with superior abilities is placed in a classroom with more severely impaired students. This may hold this student back and not enable him/her to achieve.

Some people have switched to using the international ICD-10 diagnostic system, which still has the Asperger's label. An abbreviated definition of autism in the new ICD-11 is:

- Persistent deficits in initiating and sustaining social interactions.
- Restricted, repetitive, and inflexible patterns of behavior and interests.

When this book went to press, a final draft of the ICD-11 had been published. The Asperger's label has been removed and autism is described with six levels of severity. I like the new ICD-11 draft because it provides clearer guidance. There is a heavy emphasis on whether or not the person has a disorder of intellectual development. When therapies are effective, a child or adult can progress to a higher level. Below is my simplified summary. You can access the complete ICD-11 online.

- Autism – Both without intellectual disability and normal language (formerly Asperger's diagnosis)

- Autism – Intellectual disability with normal or near-normal language.
- Autism – Without intellectual disability and with impaired functional language.
- Autism – Both impaired intellectual development and language.
- Autism – Without intellectual disability and no language.
- Autism – Intellectual disability and no language.

You Should Bust Out of the Label Silos; ADHD and Autism Overlap

Each diagnostic label has its own support group meetings and books. Unfortunately, each group may stay in its own silo and there may be little communication between them. I have observed that the books for each diagnosis are almost all particular to that diagnosis. In many cases, there are kids who fit in more than one diagnosis. There are four diagnostic labels that get mixed up all the time. They are ASD, sensory processing disorder (SPD), ADHD (attention-deficit/hyperactivity disorder), and gifted. Both the DSM-5 and ICD-11 allow a dual diagnosis of ASD and ADHD.

In fact, three studies show that there is a genetic overlap with autism and ADHD. The biggest crossover in genetic factors is between fully verbal autism (Asperger's) and ADHD. This is why autism and ADHD are often mixed up. One doctor will give a child an autism diagnosis and another will diagnose that same child as ADHD. A new neuro-imaging study shows that both autism and ADHD have similar structural abnormalities in the social parts of the brain. Some of these kids may be gifted in one academic subject and have a severe disability in another. Sometimes a child is labeled twice exceptional (or 2E) and he/she may be both gifted and have either an ASD, ADHD, or SPD diagnosis. When the same type of students get put in different silos, they often go down different paths. My observations at conferences indicate that about half the children who are brought to an autism conference are gifted in at least one area such as math, music, reading, or art. In other chapters, I will discuss the need for developing their strengths. When I attend a gifted education conference, I see the same little geeky kids going down a different, very positive path toward a career in science or art. I want to make it very clear: geek, nerd, and mild ASD are the same thing. There is a point where being socially awkward is just part of normal human variation. There is fascinating new research that shows that autism may be the price for a human brain. The same genes that make the human brain large also cause autism. Other studies have shown that autistic traits are present in the general population.

I have also given talks at many high-tech companies, and it is likely that almost half the people who work there have mild ASD. One executive at a tech company told me that he knows they have many employees with AS or mild ASD, but they don't talk about it. Many people in successful technical careers hate the ASD label because they feel that it implies that they are damaged. They avoid the labels. Recently I read about a young man who had a severe speech delay, and he was apprenticed into his father's physics lab. He had several scientific papers published before he was 20. If he had been born into a different situation, he may have taken a different path as an individual labeled with ASD.

Labels Required for School or Medical Services

Schools and insurance companies require diagnostic labels in order to get services. Unfortunately, I am seeing too many smart kids labeled ASD getting fixated on their autism. I think it would be healthier for the child to be fixated on art, writing, science, or some other special interest. Too many kids are becoming their label. When I was a student, I went to school with lots of socially awkward, geeky individuals. If DSM-5 guidelines were used, they would have been labeled autism spectrum disorder. If the new ICD-11 had been used, they would have been placed in the mildest autism category, similar to the old Asperger's diagnosis.

Both fully verbal autism and more severe ASD often look the same in nonverbal or speech-delayed children under age five. When children labeled ASD get older, they may diverge into two basic groups who need very different services. This highly divergent group is all assigned the same DSM-5 ASD label, and in poorly run programs, they are all given the same services. One group will continue to have a severe disability with either no speech or partial speech, and the other group will become fully verbal and capable of independent living and a successful career if they receive the right interventions. They usually are able to do grade-level or above-average schoolwork in at least one subject, such as reading or math.

There is a third subgroup in the nonverbal group who appear to have a severe intellectual disability. Examples of this type are Tito Mukhopadhyay and Naoki Higashida. Both of them can type independently, and they have good brains that are "locked in." From both an educational and functional standpoint, ASD becomes many different things in older children and adults. They may explain why there is so much controversy and differences of opinion in the autism community.

I am also concerned about children who should have an ASD label but they were given a label of oppositional defiant disorder (ODD) or disruptive mood dysregulation disorder (DMDD). In DMDD, the symptoms are frequent temper tantrums in a child older than six. The ODD label can be used for children of all ages. Its main symptoms are active defiance, vindictiveness, and sustained anger. Children who get these labels need to have firm limits placed on behavior and be given choices. For example, the choice could be doing homework before dinner or doing it after dinner. Choices help prevent the oppositional child from just saying "no."

In conclusion, parents and teachers must bust out of the ASD silo. DSM labels are not precise. They are behavioral profiles. Unfortunately, our system requires labels to get services. Remember to think about the specific services a child needs such as tutoring in reading, prevention of bullying, or social skills training for an older child or an intensive, early educational program for a nonverbal three-year-old.

References and Additional Reading

American Psychiatric Association (2013) *Diagnostic and Statistical Manual of Mental Disorders* (*DSM-5*) Washington, D.C.: American Psychiatric Association.

Autism Europe (2018) World Health Organization updates classification of autism in the ICD-11 www.autism.europe.org (accessed June 21, 2019).

Baribeau, D.A. et al. (2019) Structural neuroimaging correlates of social deficits are similar in autism and attention-deficit/hyperactivity disorder: Analysis from the POND Network, *Translational Psychiatry*, 4(9):72doi:10.1038/s41398-019-0392-0.

Barnett, K. (2013) *The Spark: A Mother's Story of Nurturing, Genius and Autism*, Random House, New York NY.

Constantino, J.N. et al. (2003) Autistic traits in the general population: A twin study, *Archives of General Psychology*, 60:530-534.

Grandin, T., and Panek, R. (2013) *The Autistic Brain: Thinking Across the Spectrum*, Houghton Mifflin Harcourt, New York, NY.

Grzadzinski, R., Huerta, M. and Lord, C. (2013) DSM-5 and Autism Spectrum Disorders (ASDs): An Opportunity for Identifying Subgroups, *Molecular Autism*, 4:12-13. Doi:10.1186/2040-2392-4-12.

Hazen, E., McDougle, C., and Volkmar, F. (2013) Changes in the diagnostic criteria for autism in DSM-5 controversies and concerns, *The Journal of Clinical Psychiatry*, 74:739 doi:10.4088/JCP.13ac08550.

Higashida, N. and Mitchell, D. (2017) *Fall Down Seven Times and Get Up Eight: A Young Man's Voice from the Silence of Autism*, Random House, New York NY.

May, T. et al. (2018) Trends in the overlap of autism spectrum disorders and attention deficit hyperactivity disorder, prevalence, clinical management, language and genetics, *Current Disorder Reports*, 5:49-57.

Mukhopadhyay, T. (2008) *How Can I Talk if My Lips Don't Move: Inside My Autistic Mind*, Arcade Publishing, New York NY. Amazon Kindle and Barnes & Noble Nook available. Also available as audiobook from Amazon.

Pinto, R. (2015) The genetic overlap of attention-deficit/hyperactivity disorder and autistic-like traits: An investigation of individual symptom scales and cognitive markers, *Journal of Abnormal Child Psychology* doi:10.1007/s10802-015-0037-4.

Reed, G. M. et al. (2019) Innovations and changes in the ICD-11 classification of mental behavioral and neurodevelopmental disorder, *World Psychiatry*, 18 doi:10.1002/wps.20611.

Research in Autism (2019) Autism Spectrum Disorder, Diagnostic Criteria ICD-11, www.researchautism.net (Accessed January 25, 2019).

Sikela, J.M. and Sarles-Quick, V.B. (2018) Genomic tradeoffs: Are autism and schizophrenia the steep price for a human brain? Human Genetics, 137:1-13.

Traper, A. (2018) Discoveries in the genetics of ADHD in the 21st century: New findings and implications, *American Journal of Psychiatry*, 175:943-950.

World Health Organization (2019) ICD-11, Draft, Autism Spectrum Disorder, International Classifications of Diseases, World Health Organization, Geneva, Switzerland.

Economical Quality Programs for Young Children with ASD

I was lucky to get state-of-the-art early intervention (EI) and education while growing up in the early 1950s. Despite the lack of knowledge about autism and how to treat it (aside from institutionalization, which was the norm at that time), my mother had me in an excellent speech therapy nursery school by age three and I had a nanny who spent hours and hours per week playing turn-taking games and structured, enjoyable activities with me. In addition, our household's behavior rules were welldefined and social manners and social expectations were strictly enforced. Fortunately, my parents had enough money to pay for the programs that contributed to my development and laid the foundations for successful functioning as I grew up and ventured out on my own. Adjusting the fees for inflation, the cost of my program would probably be in the mid-range, compared to early intervention programs being used today. Many programs now available are much more expensive.

Can parents on a limited budget put together a good program for their young autistic child? The answer is yes, with a little thought and planning. I have talked to parents who have put together their own successful EI program after reading a few books and enlisting the help of volunteers. Self-motivation and an unfailing desire to help their child are needed as much as education about autism. The absolute worst thing a parent can do is to let their child sit and watch TV all day or zone out unaware of his or her surroundings. This is precious time wasted, never to be regained.

Both research and practical experience have indicated that twenty or more hours of intense one-to-one interaction with an effective teacher and/or adult can kick-start speech and improve language and other behaviors in children with ASD. In many parts of the country a public school will provide only one or two hours a week of therapy with a speech therapist, an occupational therapist (OT), or a behavioral specialist. This is not enough to be really effective, but it does present an opportunity for training of the individuals who work with the child outside of the school day. This is especially true for parents, who need to take the lead and provide supplemental instruction themselves.

I recommend that parents in those situations approach the school therapists as "coaches" who can educate them about their child's autism and teach them how to do more intensive therapy at home. It also helps if family members or volunteers who are working with the child (for instance, a grandmother who has volunteered to work with a four year old) visit the school every week and watch the professional therapist work with the child. The professionals can give volunteers therapy assignments to work on with the child during the week. Invaluable information can be gleaned by watching sessions "in action" that no amount of reading will ever convey. Conversely, it might also be helpful from time to time to pay the therapist to spend an hour or two observing how the in-home program is unfolding. Sometimes a small change to a program can make a world of difference and it often takes a trained eye to spot situations like this. The weekly get-togethers are also a perfect time to discuss the child's progress and review goals and objectives for the coming week so everyone can keep track of progress and program changes.

Church and civic groups are a great place to find people who might be willing to work with a child. Other sources of help include students from the local high school or college students. When looking for volunteers to help teach the child, try to be specific about the types of things they will be doing. For instance, grandmothers might feel comfortable volunteering to "play" with a child, or help provide "simple structured, repetitive drills"—those are familiar skills most people possess. Yet the same grandmother might feel ill-equipped if you ask her to "help out with the therapeutic behavior program designed for a child with autism." Most people don't know what that type of program entails, and they may think that only someone with a college degree would have relevant skills. Be sure to mention that you (or someone else) will be providing them with basic education and training on autism to further reinforce their ability to handle what comes up. Many people are genuinely interested in helping others, provided they get some training on how to do it.

I have observed that some teachers and therapists have a knack for working with children with ASD and others do not. Passive approaches do not work. Parents need to find the people, both professionals and non-professionals, who know how to

be gently insistent, who keep the child motivated to learn, are child-centered in their approach, and are dedicated to teaching children with autism in a way they can learn, instead of insisting the child learn in the way they teach. Doing so naturally engages the child, which is the foundation of any effective program for children with autism, no matter what the cost. A useful practical book for learning teaching methods is *Autism Breakthrough* by Raun K. Kaufman.

Strategies that build on the child's area of strength and appeal to their thinking patterns will be most effective.

Different Types of Thinking in Autism

Recent studies on the brain, and especially on the brains of people diagnosed with autism spectrum disorders, are shedding light on the physiological underpinnings of our thoughts and emotions. We are gaining a better understanding of how neural pathways are formed and the extent to which biology influences behavior.

When I was much younger, I assumed that everybody perceived the world the same way I did. That is, that everybody thought in pictures. Early in my professional career, I got into a heated verbal argument with an engineer at a meat packing plant when I told him he was stupid. He had designed a piece of equipment that had flaws that were obvious to me. My visual thinking gives me the ability to do a test run in my head on a piece of equipment I've designed, just like a virtual reality computer system. Mistakes can be found prior to construction when I do this. Now I realize his problem was not stupidity, it was a lack of visual thinking. It took me years to learn that the majority of people cannot do this and that visualization skills in some people are almost nonexistent.

All minds on the autism/Asperger's spectrum are detail-oriented, but how they specialize varies. By questioning many people, both on and off the spectrum, I have learned that there are three different types of specialized thinking with crossover among these specialized thinking patterns. Determining thinking types in three-year-old children is often not possible. Dominant thinking types usually become more obvious when a child is seven to nine.

- Visual thinkers (object visualizers) think in photo-realistic pictures, like me.
- Music and math patterned thinkers (visual-spatial).
- Verbal thinkers (not visual thinkers).

Since autism is so variable, there may be mixtures of the different types. For instance, a child may have strong music/math patterned thinking, but also have good visual thinking abilities. Or a verbal thinker may also have good math or foreign language skills. The importance of understanding these three ways of thinking comes into play when trying to teach children with ASD. Strategies that build on the child's area of strength and appeal to their thinking patterns will be most effective. This is most likely to become evident between the ages of five and eight. It is often difficult to identify the strengths of children younger than five, unless savant skills are unfolding. In college students, the major they chose was partially determined by their cognitive style. Students in three different majors were assessed. Engineering students preferred visual-spatial pattern thinking. Fine arts and psychology students preferred visual thinking (object visualizer) and verbal thinking was only prominent in psychology students.

Visual Thinkers (Object Visualizers)

These children often love art and building blocks, such as Legos, and they will often produce beautiful drawings. They get easily immersed in projects that have a tangible, hands-on opportunity for learning. Math concepts, such as adding and subtracting, need to be taught starting with concrete objects the child can touch. Drawing and other art skills should be encouraged. These kids may have a really difficult time with algebra. They should be moved immediately ahead into geometry because geometry is more visual. If a child only draws one thing, such as airplanes, encourage him/her to draw other related objects, such as the airport runways, or the hangars, or cars going to the airport. Broadening a child's emerging skills helps him/her be more flexible in his/her thinking patterns. Keep in mind that because the child's "native language" is pictures, verbal responses can take longer to form. Each request has to be translated from words to pictures before it can be processed, and then the response needs to be translated from pictures into words before it is spoken. Visual thinkers often have difficulty doing algebra because of its abstract nature, but some can do geometry and trigonometry quite easily. Visual thinkers often find success in careers as artists, graphic designers, photographers, or industrial engineers. Another field visual thinkers like me can excel in is skilled trades. There is a huge shortage of plumbers, electricians, mechanics, and welders who can read blueprints. One of the worst things some schools have done was removing vocational classes. These are good careers that will never get replaced by artificial intelligence or computers.

Music and Math Thinkers (Visual-Spatial)

Patterns instead of pictures dominate the thinking processes of these children. Both music and math are a world of patterns, and children who think this way can have strong associative abilities. Research shows that they have superior abilities to perform mental rotation tasks. They like finding relationships between numbers or musical notes. Some children may have savant-type calculation skills or are able to play a piece of music after hearing it just once. Musical talent often emerges without formal instruction. Many of these children can teach themselves if instruments are available. When they grow up, pattern thinkers are often very good at computer programming, engineering, or music. Some of these children should be advanced several grades ahead in math, depending on their abilities, but they may need special education in reading which may lag behind. Many of these kids can easily do math in their heads. They should be allowed to do this. They are likely to get bored in a math class that is too easy. They also need to be exposed to computer programming and coding. One way to determine how a child thinks is to expose him/her to both algebra and geometry books.

Verbal Thinkers

These children love lists and numbers. Often, they will memorize bus timetables and events in history. Interest areas often include history, geography, weather, and sports statistics. They are not visual thinkers. Parents and teachers can use these interests and talents as motivators for learning the less interesting parts of academics. Some verbal thinkers are whizzes at learning many different foreign languages. I know individuals with verbal thinking skills who have been successfully employed in sales of specialized products such as cars, stage acting, accounting, factual/technical writing, and pharmacology. These are all areas where memorization of many facts is a talent that other people will appreciate.

The thinking patterns of individuals with ASD are markedly different from the way "normal" people think. Because of this, too much emphasis is placed on what they "can't do," and opportunities to capitalize on their different but often creative and novel ways of thinking fall by the wayside. An interesting new study showed that many students with autism who attend college enroll in STEM fields such as computer science or engineering. While impairments and challenges to exist, greater progress can be made teaching these individuals when parents and teachers work on building the child's strengths and teach in a manner aligned with their basic pattern of thinking.

References and Additional Reading

Blazhenkova, O. et al. (2011) Object-spatial imagery and verbal cognitive styles in children and adolescents: Developmental trajectories in relation to ability, *Learning and Individual Differences.*

Chiang, H.M. and Lin, Y.H. (2007) Mathematical ability of students with Asperger syndrome and high-functioning autism, *Autism* 11:547-556.

Grandin, T. (2009) How does visual thinking work in the mind of a person with autism" A personal account. *Physiological Transactions of the Royal Society*, London, UYK, 364:1437-1442.

Grandin, T. and Panek, R. (2013) *The Autistic Brain*, Houghton Mifflin Harcourt, New York, NY.

Hegarty, M., and Kozhevnikov, M. (1999) Types of visual-spatial representations and mathematical problem solving, *Journal of Educational Psychology*, 91:684-689.

Hoffner, T.N. (2016) More evidence for three kinds of cognitive styles: Validating the object-spatial imagery and verbal questionnaire using eye tracking when learning with texts and pictures, *Applied Cognitive Psychology* 31(1) doi.org/10.1002/acp.3300.

Jones, C.R.G. et al. (2009) Reading and arithmetic in adolescents with autism spectrum disorders: Peaks and dips in attainment, Neuropsychology, 23:718-728.

Kozhevnikov, M. and Blazenkova, O. (2013) Individual differences in object versus spatial imagery: From neural correlates to real world applications, In: S. Lacey and R. Lawson (Editors), Multisensory Imagery, 229-308.

Mazard, A. et al (2004) A PET meta-analysis of object and spatial mental imagery, European Journal of Cognitive Psychology 16:673-695.

Perez-Fabello, M.J. et al. (2018) Object spatial imagery in fine arts, psychology and engineering, Thinking Skills and Creativity 27:131-138.

Shonulsky, S.et al. (2019) STEM faculty experiences teaching students with autism, Journal of STEM Teacher Education 53(2) Article 4.

Resources for Computer Coding for Kids

www.scratch.mit.edu

Sphero Robots, Boulder, Colorado

www.code.org

www.codakid

www.khanacademy.org

Appled Swift Coding

Stevenson, J.L. and Gernsbacher, M.A. (2013) Abstract spatial reasoning as an autistic strength. PLOS ONE doi:10.1371/journal.pone.0059329.

McGrath, J. et al. (2012) Atypical visual spatial processing in autism: Insight from functional connectivity analysis, Autism Research, 5:314-330.

Soulieres, I. et al., (2011) The level and nature of autistic intelligence II: What about Asperger syndrome? PLOS One. Doi:10.1371/journal.pone.0025372.

Higher Expectations Yield Results

Young children with autism spectrum disorders do not learn by listening to and watching others, as do typical children.

They need to be specifically taught things that others seem to learn by osmosis. A good teacher is gently insistent with a young autistic child in order to get progress. The teacher has to be careful not to cause sensory overload, but at the same time has to be somewhat intrusive into the child's world of stimming or silent withdrawal in order for the child to engage in learning.

When children get a little older, they need to be exposed to many different things to stimulate their continued learning in different areas of life. There also need to be expectations for proper social behavior. When I look back at my life, my mother made me do a number of things I did not like, but these activities were really beneficial. They gave me opportunities to practice social skills, converse with less-familiar people, develop self-esteem and learn to negotiate unanticipated changes. None of these activities caused major problems with sensory oversensitivity. While Mother may have pushed me to do things, she understood well that a child should never be forced into a situation that includes painful sensory stimulation.

By age five, I was required to dress up and behave in church and sit through formal dinners both at home and at Granny's.

When I didn't, there was a consequence, and I lost a privilege that meant something to me. Fortunately, our church had a beautiful old-fashioned organ I liked. Most of the service was boring to me, but that organ made it somewhat tolerable to sit through. A modern church with loud, amplified music probably would be sensory overload to someone like me.

During my elementary school years, Mother had me be her party hostess. I had to greet each guest and serve them snacks. This taught me important social skills, and it made me feel proud to be participating in their "grown-up" event. It also provided the opportunity to learn how to talk to many different people.

When I was reluctant to learn to ride a bike, I was urged to learn. Mother was always testing the limits on how far she could push me. I became motivated to learn after I missed a bike trip to the Coca Cola plant.

When I was a teenager, the opportunity arose for me to visit my aunt's ranch in Arizona. At the time, I was having non-stop panic attacks and was afraid to go. Mother gave me the choice to go for two weeks or the whole summer. When I got there, I loved it and stayed all summer. Aunt Ann became one of my important mentors. My career in livestock equipment design would have never started if I had been allowed to stay home.

I often needed a certain amount of pushing to do new things by myself. I was good at building things, but afraid to go to the lumber yard and buy the wood by myself. Mother made me do it. She never let my autism be an excuse for not trying something she knew would be beneficial for me to learn. I came back crying from that outing, but I had the wood with me. Further trips to the lumber yard were easy. At one of my early jobs my boss made me "cold call" cattle magazines to get articles published. After I got over the initial fear, I found I was good at getting articles into national cattle publications. In all of the above cases, either my mother or a boss had to push me to do things even though I was afraid. Yet the things I learned—especially about myself—were priceless.

After I started my freelance design business, I almost gave it up because an early client was not 100% satisfied. My blackand-white thinking led me to believe that clients would always be 100% satisfied. Fortunately, my good friend Jim Uhl, the contractor who built my systems, would not let me quit. He actively kept pushing and talking to me and asking for the next drawing. When I produced a new drawing, he praised it. Now

I know that 100% client satisfaction is impossible. My life and career could have been derailed and wrecked if my mother and business associates had not pushed me to do things. Mother did not let me lie around the house, and never viewed my autism as rendering me incapable. Business associates stayed after me and made me do things. These adult mentors are a grown-up version of a good special education teacher who is gently insistent with a three-year-old child with autism. What it demonstrates overall is that people with ASD can learn and succeed when others around them believe in their abilities and hold high expectations of them.

To summarize this chapter, parents and teachers need to "stretch" individuals on the autism spectrum. They need to be stretched just outside their comfort zone for them to develop. However, there must be no sudden surprises, because surprises are frightening. I am seeing too many individuals with ASD who have not learned basic skills, such as shopping and shaking hands. At conferences, I see parents speaking for their child when their child should be speaking for himself. They are being overprotected and sheltered too much. It made me really happy when I encouraged a child with ASD to ask her own question in front of a whole lot of people at a conference. When the child was successful speaking in front of the crowd, the audience clapped.

Teaching Turn Taking and the Ability to Wait

I visited a school in Australia that was using simple innovative methods to teach turn taking and the ability to wait. Diane Heaney, the director of education for the AEIOU Foundation, explained the concept of this early educational program. When designing this program, she asked the question, "What are the most important things to teach children to get them ready for a mainstream first-grade class?" They are the ability to talk, take turns, sit still, exhibit good table manners, use the toilet independently, and have social engagement.

The children in her program start at age two to three years and are all nonverbal or have obviously delayed verbal skills. At the end of the three-year program, approximately 75 percent of the children have gained enough skills to go to a mainstream school. Some may need an aide or other support. The school is a full-day program, and the kids go home in the afternoon. The staff-to-student ratio is one to two.

When the children first arrive in her program, they get standard applied behavior analysis (ABA) to get language started.

After verbal skills develop, they move away from one-on-one ABA to activities that teach turn taking and the ability to wait.

Teaching Turn Taking

T hey use three different methods to teach turn taking: playing traditional board games, projecting an educational video game on a Smartboard, and sharing a tablet computer (iPad). I loved the projected video game. They used a Curious George counting game that has very distinct activities where each turn is independent (i.e., doesn't depend on the previous child's answer). Because the game is projected on a Smartboard, when each child takes his turn, the other children have to sit and watch. The Smartboard responds like a gigantic touch screen iPad. The key is having the children who wait be able to watch the child who is taking his turn to perform. This activity teaches both turn taking and sitting quietly on a chair. The projected image on the Smartboard prevents fighting over a physical tablet computer.

The following procedure is used by the teacher.

Step 1: A single child learns to play the game by himself for a few minutes and finds it rewarding.

Step 2: Two children take turns, one at a time, walking to the Smartboard and touching the screen to play a single turn of the game. The child who is waiting to take his turn must remain in his chair.

Step 3: When two children can wait and take turns, a child on a third chair is added.

Step 4: When three children can wait and take turns, a fourth child on a fourth chair is added.

If a Smartboard is not available, a tablet should be placed on a table in front of the children and each child would have to walk up and take his turn and then go back to his chair. The tablet should be positioned so that the children who are waiting can see the screen. The tablet may need to be attached to a sturdy stand so a child cannot pick it up and try to take it back to his chair. The principle is to teach the children to inhibit a response in order to get a reward. To make it easier for the other children who are waiting to watch what is happening on the tablet, the screen image could be easily projected on the wall with a standard LCD projector.

The children also have to learn how to take turns while playing traditional board games and passing a smartphone or tablet from one child to another. Teaching the children to share a phone or tablet they can hold may be more difficult. The previously described activity should be mastered first.

Remember, all school activities involving electronics with children under the age of five should always be done as an interactive activity under the supervision of a teacher. Solitary play on electronic devices must be avoided. When electronics are used, children must be interacting with either other children or an adult.

What School Is Best for My Child with ASD?

I get asked all the time by parents about which school is the best for their child with autism spectrum disorder (ASD). I have observed that success in school depends so much on the particular school and the people who are involved. Public or private is not an issue. It depends on the particular staff who work with your child. It is really important for PreK and elementary school children to get lots of contact with neurotypical children to learn appropriate social behavior.

There are many children with autism or other labels who do really well in their local public school system and are mainstreamed in a regular classroom. Children who have been successfully mainstreamed range from fully verbal advanced placement (AP) students to students who are nonverbal and/or are more severely involved. Unfortunately, there are other schools that are doing poorly due to a variety of factors.

Some parents choose to homeschool their child. There are lots of good homeschooling materials on the Internet, such as Khan Academy (*www.khanacademy.org*), which offers a multitude of free classroom materials for math and science. Others look for a special school for their spectrum kid.

Special Schools for ASD

Recently I toured specialized schools for both elementary and high school students who are on the spectrum. Within the last few years, many new specialized schools have opened. They tend to fall into two types. One is designed for fully verbal children who have autism, Asperger's, attention deficit hyperactivity disorder (ADHD), dyslexia, or some other learning problem. The kids are enrolled in their new school to get away from being bullied or to keep from becoming lost in the crowd in a huge school. The other type of special school is designed to fit the needs of students who are nonverbal and/or have challenging behaviors.

I have visited four-day schools that enroll children with autism or other labels who just do not fit in at a regular school. Teasing and bullying were often a major reason for leaving the former school. Problems with aggression in many students on the spectrum disappeared when the teasing stopped. None of these schools accepted kids who had been in serious trouble with the law. Most of the students I met at these schools were fully verbal and did not have serious problems, such as self injurious behavior. They were kids who were a lot like me when I was their age. The student population ranged from 30 to 150.

Keeping the schools small is one of the keys to the success of these special ASD schools.

Effective Classrooms for ASD

I observed two types of classrooms at these specialized schools. The first type was just like my old 1950s–style elementary school. There were about 12 children in each class, and they all sat at desks while the teacher taught in the front of the classroom.

Keeping classes small was essential. The school enrolled about 100 students, ranging from kindergarten through high school. These students were mainly the socially awkward geeky kids who got picked on by bullies. I talked to them at an assembly where all the students sat on the floor of the gym, and their behavior was wonderful!

The other type of classroom I observed had a teacher to student ratio of 1:3 or 1:4. Students from several different grades were in the same classroom, and students were taught in subject areas such as math, science, or English. Each student worked at his own pace as the teacher rotated among the students. In all the classrooms a quiet environment was maintained because many students have difficulty with sensory issues. I was glad to see that in most of the classrooms hands-on activities were used.

Every child is different. What works for one may not work for another. There is also a lot of variation in schools, from city to city, and region to region. You know your child best. Take into account your child's strengths and challenges when deciding the right school for him to find the best possible match. Most importantly, make sure the staff at the school have the proper training and background and use instructional methods that are a good fit for your child's needs.

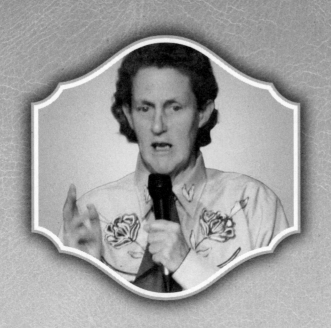

CHAPTER 2

Teaching & Education

Good teachers understand that for a child to learn, the teaching style must match the student's learning style.

E very child with ASD has his or her own personality and profile of strengths and weaknesses; this is no different than with typical children. They can be introverts or extroverts, have a sunny disposition or be cranky, love music or math. Parents and educators can easily forget this, and attribute every action or reaction of the child to autism or Asperger's, and therefore in need of dissection and "fixing." The goal in teaching children with autism is not to turn them into clones of their typical peers (i.e., "normal"). When you think about it, not all characteristics exhibited by typical people are worthy of being modeled. A much more meaningful perspective is to teach this population the academic and interpersonal skills they need to be *functional* in the world and use their talents to the best of their ability.

Autism is not a death sentence for a child or the family. It brings with it great challenges, but it can also bring to the child the seeds of great talents and unique abilities. It is the responsibility of parents and educators to find those seeds, nurture them, and make sure they grow. That should be the goal of teaching and education for children with ASD too, not just for typical children.

The different thinking patterns of individuals with ASD require parents and educators to teach from a new frame of reference, one aligned with their autism way of thinking. Expecting children with ASD to learn via the conventional curriculum and teaching methods that "have always worked" for typical children is to set everyone up for failure right from the start. It would be like placing a young child on a grown up's chair and expecting his feet to reach the floor. That's just silly, isn't it? Yet, surprisingly, that is still how many schools and educators approach students with ASD. Good teachers understand that for a child to learn, the teaching style must match the student's learning style. With autism and especially with Asperger's students, it is not enough to match the teaching style to the child's learning type.

Educators must take this idea one step further, and be continuously mindful that students with ASD come to school without a developed social thinking framework. This is the aspect of ASD that can be difficult for adults to understand, envision, and work around. Our public education system is built upon the premise that children enter school with basic social functioning skills in place. Kids with autism—with their characteristic social thinking challenges—enter school already lagging far behind their classmates. Teachers who don't recognize this and don't make accommodations to teach social thinking and social skills alongside traditional academics just further limit the opportunities children with ASD have to learn and grow.

To Mainstream or Not to Mainstream?

At age five I started attending a small school with typical children. In today's language, that would be called mainstreaming. It is important to note that this worked for me because the structure and composition of the class was well matched to my needs. The school had highly structured old-fashioned classes with only twelve students. Children were expected to behave and there were strict rules, enforced consistently, and with consequences applied for infractions. The environment was relatively quiet and controlled, without a high degree of sensory stimulation. In this environment I did not need an aide. Contrast that classroom with today's learning environment. In a class of thirty students, with a single teacher, in a less structured classroom within a larger school, I would never have survived without the direct assistance of a one-on-one aide.

Whether or not to mainstream an elementary school child on the autism spectrum is a decision that should take many factors into consideration. After countless discussions with parents and teachers, I have come to the conclusion that much depends on the particular school and the particular teachers in that school. The idea of mainstreaming is a worthy goal, and in an ideal situation—where all the variables are working in favor of the child with ASD—it can be a highly positive experience. But the reality of the situation is often the opposite: lack of teacher training, large classes, limited opportunities for individual modifications, and lack of funding to support one-on-one paraprofessionals can render this environment disastrous for the spectrum child.

For elementary school children on the higher functioning end of the autism spectrum, I usually favor mainstreaming because it is essential for them to learn social skills from typically developing children. If a child is homeschooled or goes to a special school, it is imperative that the child has regular engagement with typical peers. For nonverbal children, mainstreaming works well in some situations—again, much depends on the school, its expertise in autism, and its program. A special school may be a better choice for the nonverbal or cognitively impaired child with autism, especially in cases where severe, disruptive behavior problems exist and need to be addressed.

Parents frequently ask me whether or not they should change the school or program their child is in. My response is to ask this question: "Is your child making progress and improving where he is now?" If they say he is, I usually recommend staying in the school or the program and then discuss whether some additional services or program modifications may be needed. For instance, the child may do even better with more attention to physical exercise, or addressing his sensory problems, or adding a few more hours of individualized ABA (Applied Behavior Analysis) therapy or social skills training.

However, if the child is making little or no progress, and the school's attitude is not supportive or accommodating of the different needs and learning styles of children with ASD so the parent is constantly battling for even the most basic services, it may be best to find a different school or program. This will, of course, require time and effort on the part of the parent, but it is important for parents to keep the end goal in sight—giving the child as much opportunity to learn and acquire needed skills in as supportive an environment as possible.

It does no one good, and least of all the child, for a parent to repeatedly fight a school system, either within IEP meetings or through due process, to win their case within an environment of individuals who are not interested in truly helping the child.

Sadly, this scenario plays out in schools and districts across the country. Valuable time that could be spent in meaningful instruction that helps the child is wasted while the school and parent butt heads for not just months, but in many cases, years. The child—and the child's needs—should always remain the focus. If the school is not child-focused, then parents should find one that is.

I reiterate a point made earlier: so much depends on the *particular people* working with the child. In one case, a third grader in a good school with an excellent reputation had several teachers who simply did not like him, nor did they attempt to understand his learning style and modify instruction to meet that style. The child hated going to school. I suggested the parents try to find a different school. They did, and the child is now doing great in his new school. In my conversations with parents and teachers, I have also observed that it doesn't matter whether the elementary school is public or private; this is seldom the issue. More depends on local conditions: the school's perception of children with disabilities and philosophy towards their education, the extent to which staff have been trained/receive ongoing training on autism spectrum disorders and how best to work with this population, and the support provided by administration to staff in educating these students. Decisions must be made on a case-by-case basis.

The Parent Guilt Trip

It is unfortunate, but a reality of today's society, that some individuals and companies who run special schools, sell therapy services, or market products to the autism community often try to put parents on a guilt trip. All parents want what's best for their child, and parents of newly diagnosed children can be especially vulnerable. These vendors prey upon parents' emotions in advertising and personal encounters, suggesting that parents are not good parents if they don't try their program or product, or that by not using whatever it is they offer, the parent isn't doing "everything possible" to help their child. Some go as far as to tell parents that their child is doomed unless they use their program or product.

One parent called me about a situation just like this. The family was ready to sell their house to have the funds needed to send their four-year-old child with autism to a special school in another state. I asked him if the child was learning and making progress at the local public school. The dad told me he was. Yet, the special school was making great claims about the progress their child would make with them. I talked with the dad about the negative impact disrupting the child's life like this might have, taking him away from his family and familiar surroundings, and sending him to a school in another state. The very real possibility existed that the child could get worse, rather than better. By the time we ended our conversation, the parents decided to keep their child in his local school and supplement his education with some additional hours of one-to-one therapy.

The articles in this section shed light on the different thinking and learning patterns of children with ASD. They offer many teaching tips to help children succeed. Among the different topics covered are areas that I view as especially important: developing the child's strengths, using a child's obsessions to motivate schoolwork, and teaching the child problem-solving and thinking skills that will assist him not just during his limited years in school, but throughout his entire life.

Teachable Moments

When I was a child in the 1950's, manners and social skills were taught to all children in a more structured and systematic manner. This was extremely helpful for me and for many people of my generation who were on the milder end of the autism spectrum. When I was in college, I had several friends who today would have been labeled with autism. My friends who were raised much like I was, acquired and retained good jobs.

Parents in the 1950's constantly used "teachable moments" to teach manners. Every day there will be many teachable moments. The big mistake many parents and teachers make when a child does something wrong is to scream "No." A better technique is to give the instruction instead. For example, if the child eats mashed potatoes with his hands say, "Use the fork." If I forgot to say "please" or "thank you," mother would cue me and say, "You forgot to say _____ and wait for me to respond." If I touched items in a store, she would say, "Put it back. You only touch things you will be buying." You always give instructions on how to behave.

Books That Give Insight into Autistic Thinking & Learning Patterns

Grandin, T. (2005). *Unwritten Rules of Social Relationships: Decoding Social Mysteries Through the Unique Perspectives of Autism.* Arlington, TX: Future Horizons, Inc.

Grandin T. (2006). *Thinking in Pictures* (Expanded Edition). New York: Vintage Press/Random House.

Tammet D. (2007). *Born on a Blue Day: Inside the Extraordinary Mind of an Autistic Savant.* New York: Free Press.

Grandin, T. and Panek , R. (2013). *The Autistic Brain.* Houghton Mifflin Harcourt, New York, NY.

Most individuals on the spectrum have areas of strength that can be nurtured and developed into marketable employment skills.

Finding a Child's Area of Strength

I n one of my 2005 columns in the *Autism Asperger's Digest*, I discussed the three different types of specialized thinking in individuals with high functioning autism and Asperger's Syndrome (HFA/AS). Children on the spectrum usually have an area of strength and an area of deficit. Many parents and teachers have asked me, "How do you determine the child's area of strength?" A child usually has to be at least in elementary school before it becomes evident. In many cases, the area of strength cannot be determined in a child younger than five years old. In some cases the area of strength doesn't emerge until some of the other, more dominant sensory or behavioral issues have been remediated.

The first type is the visual thinkers, who think in photorealistic pictures. I am in this category, and my mind works like Google Images. When I was in elementary school, my visual thinking skills were expressed in art and drawing. Children who are visual thinkers will usually produce many beautiful drawings by the time they are in third or fourth grade. In my career, I use my visual thinking skills to design livestock-handling facilities. Visual thinkers often go into such careers as graphic arts, industrial design, or architecture.

The second type is the pattern thinkers, who are often very good at math and music. They see relationships and patterns between numbers and sounds. In elementary school, some of these children will play a musical instrument really well. Others will be good at both music and math, and another group will be math lovers with no musical interest. It is important to challenge these kids with advanced math. If they are forced to do "baby" math, they will get bored. If an elementary school student can do high school math, he or she should be encouraged to study it. Both photo-realistic visual thinkers and pattern thinkers often excel at building structures with blocks and Legos®. Pattern thinkers can have successful careers as engineers, computer programmers or musicians. However, the pattern thinkers will often need some extra help with reading and writing composition.

The third type is the verbal thinker. These children are word specialists and they know all the facts about their favorite subjects. For many of these kids, history is their favorite subject and their writing skills are good. The word thinkers are not visual thinkers and they will usually have little interest in art, drawing, or Legos. Individuals who are word specialists are often really good at journalism, being speech therapists, and any job that requires careful record keeping.

Build Up Strengths

Too often educators pound away at the deficits and neglect to build up the child's area of strength. Most visual thinkers and some pattern thinkers cannot do algebra. Algebra was impossible for me, and therefore, I was never allowed to try geometry or trigonometry. Endless hours of algebra drills were useless. I did not understand it because there was nothing to visualize. When I discuss this at conferences, I find many children and adults on the spectrum who failed algebra, but were able to do geometry and trigonometry. They should be allowed to substitute these higher maths for algebra. Algebra is NOT the prerequisite for geometry and trigonometry for some types of brains.

Educators need to understand that these individuals think differently and that what works for the typical-minded student may not work for the spectrum individual. I got through college math because in the '60s, algebra had been replaced with finite math, where I studied probability and matrices. It was difficult but with tutoring I was able to do it. Finite math had things I could visualize. If I had been forced to take college algebra, I would have failed college math. Students should be allowed to substitute any higher math for algebra. One mother told me her son got straight As in college physics but he could not graduate from high school because he failed algebra.

One of the worst things many schools have done is removing classes such as art, sewing, band, auto repair, welding, music, theater, and other "hands on" classes. In elementary school, I would have been lost without art, sewing, and woodworking class. These were the classes where I had strengths and I learned skills that became the basis of my work on design and livestock facilities.

In conclusion, focusing only on the deficits of individuals with HFA/AS does nothing to prepare them for the real world that lies outside of school. Most individuals on the spectrum have areas of strength that can be nurtured and developed into marketable employment skills. Teachers and parents need to build on these areas of strength starting when the child is young, and continue through middle and high school. In so doing, we provide these individuals with the opportunity to have satisfying careers they can enjoy for the rest of their lives.

Teachers and parents need to help both children and adults with autism ta e all the little details they have in their head and put them into categories to form concepts and promote generalization.

Teaching How to Generalize

M any children and people with autism are not able to take all the facts they know and link them together to form concepts. What has worked for me is to use my visual thinking to form concepts and categories. Explaining how I do this may help parents and professionals teach children with autism how to form concepts and generalizations.

When I was a little child, I knew that cats and dogs were different because dogs were bigger than cats. When the neighbors bought a little Dachshund, I could no longer categorize dogs by size. Rosie the Dachshund was the same size as a cat. I can remember looking intently at Rosie to find some visual characteristic that both our Golden Retriever and Rosie had in common.

I noticed that all dogs, regardless of size, had the same kind of nose. Therefore, dogs could be placed in a separate category from cats because there are certain physical features that every dog has that no cat has.

Categorizing things can be taught. Little kindergarten children learn to categorize all the red objects or all the square objects. Irene Pepperberg, a scientist at the University of Arizona, taught her parrot, Alex, to differentiate and identify objects by color and shape. He could pick out all the red square blocks from a tray containing red balls, blue square blocks, and red blocks. He understood categorization of objects by color, shape, and size. Teaching children and adults with autism to categorize and form concepts starts first with teaching simple categories such as color and shape. From this, we can help them understand that certain facts they have memorized can be placed in one category and other facts can be placed in another category.

Teaching Concepts Such as Danger

Many parents have asked me, "How do I teach my child not to run into the street?" or "He knows not to run into the street at our house, but at Grandma's he runs into the street." In the first situation, the child actually has no concept of danger at all; in the second, he is not able to generalize what he has learned at home to a new house and street.

Danger as a concept is too abstract for the mind of a person who thinks in pictures. I did not understand that being hit by a car would be dangerous until I saw a squashed squirrel in the road and my nanny told me that it had been run over by a car. Unlike the cartoon characters on TV, the squirrel did not survive. I then understood the cause and effect of being run over.

After the squirrel incident, how did I learn that all cars on all streets are dangerous? It is just like learning concepts like the color red or square versus round. I had to learn that no matter where I was located, all cars and all streets had certain common features. When I was a child, safety concepts were drilled into my head with a book of safety songs. I sang about always looking both ways before crossing a street to make sure a car was not coming. To help me generalize, my nanny took my sister and me for walks around the neighborhood. On many different streets she had me look both ways before crossing. This is the same way that guide dogs for the blind are trained. The dog must be able to recognize stop lights, intersections, and streets in a strange place. During training, he is taken to many different streets. He then has visual, auditory and olfactory (smell) memories of many different streets. From these memories, the dog is able to recognize a street in a strange place.

For either the guide dog or the person with autism to understand the concept of street, they have to see more than one street. Autistic thinking is specific to general. To learn a concept of *dog* or *street*, I had to see many specific dogs or streets before the general concept could be formed. A general concept such as street without pictures of many specific streets stored in my memory bank is absolutely meaningless.

Autistic thinking is always detailed and specific. Teachers and parents need to help both children and adults with autism take all the little details they have in their head and put them into categories to form concepts and promote generalization.

Interests and talents can turn into careers.

The Importance of Developing Talent

There is often too much emphasis in the world of autism on the deficits of these children and not enough emphasis on developing the special talents that many of them possess. Talents need to be developed because they can form the basis of skills that will make a person with autism or Asperger's employable.

Abilities such as drawing or math skills need to be nurtured and expanded. The abilities may not become fully apparent until the child is seven or eight. If a child likes to draw trains, that interest should be broadened into other activities, such as reading a book about trains or doing a math problem calculating the time it would take to travel from Boston to Chicago.

It is a mistake to stamp out a child's special interests, however odd they may seem at the time. In my own case, my talent in art was encouraged. My mother bought me professional art materials and a book on perspective drawing when I was in grade school.

Fixations and special interests should be directed into constructive channels instead of being abolished to make a person more "normal." The career I have today as a designer of livestock facilities is based on my talent areas. I use my visual thinking to design equipment. As a teenager, I became fixated on cattle squeeze chutes after I discovered that when I got in a cattle squeeze chute it relieved my anxiety. Fixations can be great motivators if they are properly channeled. My high school teacher directed my interest in cattle chutes into motivating me to study science and to study more in school. He told me that if I learned more about the field of sensory perception, I could find out why the pressure applied by the cattle chute was relaxing. Now, instead of boring everybody I knew with endless talk about cattle chutes, I immersed myself in the study of science. My original interest in the cattle chute also led to an interest in the behavior of cattle, then the design of systems, which led to the development of my career.

This is an example of taking a fixation and broadening it out into something constructive. Sometimes teachers and parents put so much emphasis on making a teenager more social that developing talents is neglected. Teaching social skills is very important, but if the person with autism is stripped of all their special interests, they may lose meaning in their life. "I am what I think and do, more than what I feel." Social interactions can be developed through shared interests. I had friends as a child because other children liked making craft projects with me.

During the difficult years of high school, special interest clubs can be a lifesaver.

Recently I watched a TV documentary about autism. One of the people profiled liked to raise chickens. Her life took on meaning when she discovered that other people shared the same hobby. When she joined a poultry hobby club, she received social recognition for being an expert.

Interests and talents can turn into careers. Developing and nurturing these unique abilities can make life more fulfilling for a person with autism.

Teaching People on the Autism Spectrum to Be More Flexible

R igidity in both behavior and thinking is a major characteristic of people with autism and Asperger's. They have difficulty understanding the concept that sometimes it is okay to break a rule. I heard about a case where an autistic boy had a severe injury but he did not leave the school bus stop to get help.

He had been taught to stay at the bus stop so that he would not miss the bus; he could not break that rule. Common sense would have told most people that getting help for a severe injury would be more important than missing the bus. But not to this young man.

How can common sense be taught? I think it starts with teaching flexible thinking at a young age. Structure is good for children with autism, but sometimes plans can, and need to be, changed. When I was little, my nanny made my sister and me do a variety of activities. This variety prevented rigid behavior patterns from forming. I became more accustomed to changes in our daily or weekly routines and learned that I could still manage when change occurred. This same principle applies to animals. Cattle that are always fed from the red truck by Jim may panic if Sally pulls up in a white truck to feed them. To prevent this problem, progressive ranchers have learned to alter routines slightly so that cattle learn to accept some variation.

Another way to teach flexible thinking is to use visual metaphors, such as mixing paint. To understand complex situations, such as when occasionally a good friend does something nasty, I imagine mixing white and black paint. If the friend's behavior is mostly nice, the mixture is a very light gray; if the person is really not a friend then the mixture is a very dark gray. Black-and-white thinking on concepts such as "good" and "bad" can be a problem. There are degrees of badness that can be ranked in categories by severity, i.e., 1) stealing a pen, 2) punching another person, 3) robbing a bank, and 4) murder.

Flexibility can also be taught by showing the person with autism that categories can change. Objects can be sorted by color, function, or material. To test this idea, I grabbed a bunch of black, red, and yellow objects in my office and laid them on the floor. They were a stapler, a roll of tape, a ball, videotapes, a toolbox, a hat, and pens. Depending upon the situation, any of these objects could be used for either work or play. Ask the child to give concrete examples of using a stapler for work or play. For instance, stapling office papers is work; stapling a kite together is play. Simple situations like this that teach a child flexibility in thinking and relating can be found numerous times in each day.

Children do need to be taught that some rules apply everywhere and should not be broken. To teach an autistic child to not run across the street, he has to be taught the rule in many different places; the rule has to be generalized and part of that process is making sure the child understands that the rule should not be broken. However, there are times when an absolute adherence to the rule can cause harm. Children also need to be taught that some rules can change depending on the situation. Emergencies are one such category where rules may be allowed to be broken.

Parents, teachers, and therapists can continually teach and reinforce flexible thinking patterns in children with autism/AS. I hope I have provided some ideas on how to do this while still accommodating the visual manner in which they think.

Teaching Concepts to Children with Autism

Generally, people with autism possess good skills in learning rules, but they can have less developed abstract thinking skills. Dr. Nancy Minshew and her colleagues at the University of Pittsburgh have done research that may help teachers understand how the autistic mind thinks. For the autistic, learning rules is easy, but learning flexibility in thinking is difficult, and must be taught.

There are three basic levels of conceptual thinking: 1) learning rules, 2) identifying categories, and 3) inventing new categories. Category forming ability can be tested by placing a series of objects on a table, such as pencils, notepads, cups, nail files, paper clips, napkins, bottles, videotapes, and other common objects. A person with autism can easily identify all the pencils, or all the bottles. He can also easily identify objects in simple categories, such as all the objects that are green or all the metal objects. Conceptual thinking at this basic level is generally not a problem.

Where the person with autism has extreme difficulty is inventing new categories, which is the beginning of true concept formation. For example, many of the objects in the list referenced above could be classified by use (i.e., office supplies) or by shape (round/not round). To me, it is obvious that a cup, a bottle, and a pencil are all round. Most people would classify a video cassette as not-round; however, I might put it into the round category because of its round spools inside.

One of the easiest ways to teach concept formation is through playing category-forming games with children. For example, a cup can be used to drink from, or to store pencils or paper clips. In one situation, it is used for drinking; in the other, it is used in the office or at work. A videotape can be used for recreation or education, depending on the content of the tape. Notepads can be used for note taking, for art drawings, or, more abstractly, as a paperweight or a coaster for a glass. Activities such as these must be done with a high degree of repetition; it will take some time for the person with autism to learn to think differently. However, with perseverance, results will occur.

Helping children "get into their head" different and varied ways of categorizing objects is the first step in developing flexible thinking. The more examples provided, the more flexible his or her thinking can become. The more flexible the thinking, the easier it will be for the person with autism to learn to develop new categories and concepts. Once the child has acquired some flexible thinking skills with concrete objects, teachers can begin to expand their conceptual thinking into the less concrete areas of categorizing feelings, emotions, facial expressions, etc.

Flexible thinking is a highly important ability that is often—to the detriment of the child—omitted as a teachable skill on a child's IEP. It impacts a child in all environments, both now and in the future: school, home, relationships, employment, recreation. Parents and teachers need to give it more attention when developing a child's educational plan.

Reference

Minshew, N.J., J. Meyer, and G. Goldstein. 2002. Abstract reasoning in autism: a dissociation between concept formation and concept identification. *Neurospychology* 16: 327-334.

Bottom-Up Thinking and Learning Rules

Individuals on the autism spectrum learn to form concepts by grouping many specific examples of a particular concept into a virtual "file folder" in their brain. There may be a file folder labeled "Dogs," full of many mental pictures of different kinds of dogs—together, all those mental pictures form a concept of "Dog." A person on the autism spectrum may have many of these virtual file folders in their brain—one for each different concept (rudeness, turn-taking, street safety, etc.). As a person grows older, they create new file folders and add new pictures to the ones in their old file folders.

People on the autism spectrum think differently from non autistic, or "typical" people. They are "bottom-up," or "specific-to-general" thinkers. For example, they may need to see many, many different kinds of dogs before the concept of dog is permanently fixed in their mind. Or they may need to be told many times, in many places, that they must stop, look, and listen before crossing the street before the concept of street safety is permanently fixed in their mind. People on the spectrum create the concepts of dog, street safety, and everything else by "building" them from many specific examples.

Non-autistic, or "typical" people think in a completely different way. They are "top-down thinkers," or "general-to-specific" thinkers. They form a concept first, and then add in specific details. For example, they already have a general concept of what a dog looks like, and as they see more and more dogs, they add the details of what all kinds of different dogs (poodles, basset hounds, dachshunds, etc.) look like. Once someone tells them to stop, look, and listen before crossing the street, they know to do this at every street, in every neighborhood.

Bottom-up learning can be used to teach both very concrete and more abstract concepts ranging from basic safety rules to reading comprehension. In this article I will give examples starting from the most concrete concepts and finishing with more abstract ones. All concepts, regardless of the level of abstraction, must be taught with many *specific examples* for each concept.

To teach a basic safety rule, such as not running across the street, it must be taught in more than one place. This is required to make the safety rule "generalize" to new places. It must be taught at the street at home, at streets near the school, at the next-door neighbor's house, at streets around grandmother's house, or Aunt Georgia's house, and when the child visits a new, strange place. The number of different specific examples required will vary from child to child. When I was little, I was taught turn-taking with a board game called Parcheesi. If my turn-taking lessons had been limited to this game they would not have generalized to other situations, such as taking turns with my sister to use a sled or a toy. During all of these activities, I was told I had to take turns. Turn-taking in conversation was also taught at the dining room table. If I talked too long, Mother told me I had to give someone else a turn to talk.

Using many specific examples should also be used for teaching number concepts. To achieve generalization, a child should be taught counting, adding, and subtracting, with many different kinds of objects. You can use cups, candies, toy dinosaurs, pens, Matchbox cars, and other things to teach the abstract idea that arithmetic applies to many things in the real world. For example $5 - 2 = 3$ can be taught with five candies. If I eat 2 of them, I have 3 left. To learn concepts such as less and more, or fractions, try using cups of water filled to different levels, cutting up an apple, and cutting up cardboard circles. If you only used cardboard circles, the child might think that the concept of fractions applies only to cardboard circles. To teach bigger versus smaller, use different-sized objects such as bottles, candies, shirts, blocks, toy cars, and other things.

More Abstract Concepts

To move up a degree in the abstractness of concepts, I will give some examples for teaching concepts such as "up" and "down." Again, you must use many specific examples to teach these concepts.

The squirrel is "up" in the tree.

The stars are "up" in the sky.

We throw the ball "up" in the air.

We slide "down" the slide.

We dig a hole "down" in the ground.

We bend "down" to tie our shoes.

To fully comprehend the concept, the child needs to participate in the activity while the parent or teacher says a short sentence containing the word "up" or "down." Be sure to vocally emphasize the concept word. If the child has difficulty with verbal language, combine the word with a picture card that says "up" or "down."

Recently I was asked, "How did you comprehend the concept of rude behavior or good table manners?" Concepts that relate to judgments or social expectations are much more abstract for a child, yet they can still be taught in the same way. When I did something that was bad table manners, such as waving my fork in the air, Mother explained to me—very simply and without a lot of verbal chatter—that it was bad table manners. "Temple, waving your fork in the air is bad table manners." She used many naturally occurring teachable moments, helping me connect my action to the concept "bad table manners." She did this matter-of-factly and kept the message simple and consistent. Learning many specific examples also worked when she taught me the concept of rudeness. When I did something that was rude, such as belching or cutting in line, Mother told me I was being rude. Gradually a "rude" concept formed in my brain from the many specific examples.

Reading Comprehension

Many children on the spectrum can decode and read, but they have problems with comprehension. To start, focus on the very concrete facts, such as characters' names, cities they visited, or activities they did, such as playing golf. This is generally easier for the child to comprehend. Then move on to more abstract concepts in a passage of literature. For example, if they read, "Jim ate eggs and bacon" they may have difficulty answering the multiple-choice question: "Did Jim eat breakfast, lunch, or dinner?" Teach the child to break apart the question and scan his or her brain files for information that may help with comprehension. For instance, I would search through the files in my brain for pictures of meals. A picture of eggs with bacon is the best match for breakfast compared to lunch and dinner pictures.

These more abstract concepts and associations don't develop quickly. The child will need to add more and more information into his brain computer before he can be successful with abstractions. This data comes from experiences, which is why parents and teachers need to give the child lots and lots of opportunities for repetitive practice on a concept or lesson. I would start to learn this sort of concept only after a teacher had explained many different stories to me.

Laying the Foundation for Reading Comprehension

P arents and teachers of children on the autism spectrum tell me all the time that their child or student can read really well but lacks comprehension. This column outlines some of my ideas for laying the foundation for good reading comprehension.

Start with the Concrete

To teach reading comprehension, start with concrete (fact-based) questions about the information in a short story or article. Concrete questions are literal and have a correct answer. Some examples of a concrete question based on a short story about Jane's winter day are "What color is Jane's coat?" or "What town does Jane live in?" Words that would answer these, such as "red" or "Milltown," can be answered from details in the text.

Mix in Abstract Questions

After the student is successful at answering a variety of concrete comprehension questions, progress to asking slightly more abstract questions about a short story. These questions require comprehension of more general concepts. For example, "Jane and Jim went to the store. Jane bought a necklace, and Jim bought a shirt." The question could be, "Did Jim buy clothing?"

An even more abstract level of comprehension is illustrated in a question about the following sentences. "Jim is going on an expedition to

Antarctica. The weather is extremely cold there." The question could be, "Will Jim need winter clothes?"

Provide a Variety of Examples

Many children and adults with autism are not able to take all the facts they know and link them together to form concepts. However, they do excel at recognizing individual facts and details. Parents and teachers can use this strength to build reading comprehension.

Bottom-up thinkers learn to generalize and develop concepts by first recognizing details or specific examples, collecting these in their heads, and then putting them into a category to form a concept. This mental process is similar to putting scraps of related information into a common file.

Children need to be exposed to many different examples of a general or abstract concept, both in reading and in real-life experiences. For example, my concept of danger (from cars in the street) was formed from seeing a squirrel that had been run over by a car, and this example was followed by many other examples of danger connected to fast-moving vehicles.

Deconstruct Complexity

The same principle applies for more complex reading texts. Comprehension can be taught gradually by pointing out many specific examples that illustrate the larger concept. In college, I called this process "finding the basic principle." I never forgot the concepts my English literature professor taught on deriving meaning from complicated classics. I found his description of Shakespeare, Homer, and other authors super interesting.

In longer reading materials, such as a chapter in a book, the child will need to be able to identify and answer questions about the main idea. The teacher could have the child read passages from a book and then dissect the chapter in a methodical manner for the child so that he understands how the *main idea* is derived. After the teacher explains the concept the author is conveying, the student will start to understand the concept of finding the main idea of other reading materials. Repeat this process with several other texts to provide the student with ample examples of identifying the main idea.

To help a student understand an author's *opinion*, a teacher could start with editorials in a newspaper or online publication and then point by point explain how the gist of the author's opinion is determined. For example, an editorial in a local newspaper may be informing citizens of a potential dog park. The author describes the pros and cons of having a dog park, and the student could be guided to categorize each of the author's points under pro and con headings. The comprehension question could be, "Is the author in favor or not in favor of starting a dog park?"

Deconstruct Complexity

Teacher: Break down complex ideas, main points, and emotional content into smaller examples or details so student can gather this information into one larger conceptual file.

Student: Make judgments, "read between the lines," and evaluate emotional content.

Provide a Variety of Examples

Teacher: Use the strengths of bottomup thinkers to perceive the details.

Student: Build from examples to single concept.

Mix in Abstract Questions

Teacher: Progress to asking abstract questions about information in a short story.

Student: Make associations, generalize, and draw inferences.

Start with the Concrete

Teacher: Start with concrete questions about factual information in a short story.

Student: Answer concrete (factbased) questions, based on details, where a right or wrong answer exists.

It would be best to start by choosing reading materials where the author's opinion is easy to determine, and then gradually move toward texts where the author's opinion is more nuanced. After several examples, the student should start understanding how to identify an author's opinion.

Another level of complexity is understanding the *emotional content* of text. The best way to teach this is to take a variety of reading materials and step by step explain how to determine emotional content. An example of emotional content would be, "Jim was smiling and laughing at silly stunts on a reality show." The question could be, "Was Jim happy or sad?"

Regardless of the level of abstraction, reading for comprehension should be taught with many specific examples. How many examples needed will differ for each individual. Teachers and parents can help by giving many opportunities for repetitive practice. Incorporating the bottom-up approach in teaching will give the student time to build a mental file of examples to use when analyzing future reading materials.

Motivating Students

One frequent characteristic of individuals on the autism/Asperger's spectrum is an obsessive interest in one or a few particular subjects, to the exclusion of others. These individuals may be near-genius on a topic of interest, even at a very early age. Parents have described to me their ten-year-old child whose knowledge of electricity rivals that of a college senior, or a near-teen whose knowledge of insects far surpasses that of his biology teacher. However, as motivated as they are to study what they enjoy, these students are often equally unmotivated when it comes to schoolwork outside their area of interest.

It was like this with me when I was in high school. I was totally unmotivated about schoolwork in general. But I was highly motivated to work on the things that interested me, such as showing horses, painting signs, and doing carpentry projects. Luckily, my mother and some of my teachers used my special interests to keep me motivated. Mr. Carlock, my science teacher, took my obsessive interests in cattle chutes and the squeeze machine to motivate me to study science.

The squeeze machine relaxed me. Mr. Carlock told me that if I really wanted to know why the machine had this effect, I would have to study the boring school subjects so that I could graduate and then go to college to become a scientist who could answer this question. Once I really grasped the idea that to get from here to there—from middle school to graduation to college and then to a job of interest to me—I needed to apply myself to all my school subjects, boring or not. This understanding maintained my motivation to complete the work.

While students are in elementary school, teachers can easily keep them involved by using a special interest to motivate their learning. An example would be taking a student's interest in trains and using a train theme in many different subjects. In history class, read about the history of the railroad; in math class, involve trains in problem solving; in science class, discuss different forms of energy that trains utilized then and now, etc.

As students move into middle and high school, they can get turned on by visiting interesting workplaces, such as a construction site, an architecture firm, or a research lab. This makes the idea of a career real to the student and they begin to understand the education path they must take early on in school to achieve that career. If visiting a work site is not possible, invite parents who have interesting jobs into the school classroom to talk with students about their jobs. Lots of pictures to show what the work is like are strongly recommended. This is also an opportunity for students to hear about the social side of employment, which can provide motivation for making new friends, joining groups or venturing out into social situations that might be uncomfortable at first.

Students on the spectrum need to be exposed to new things in order to become interested in them. They need to see concrete examples of really cool things to keep them motivated to learn.

I became fascinated by optical illusions after seeing a single movie in science class that demonstrated optical illusions. My science teacher challenged me to recreate two famous optical illusions, called the Ames Distorted Room and the Ames Trapezoidal Window. I spent six months making them out of cardboard and plywood and I finally figured them out. This motivated me to study experimental psychology in college.

Bring Trade Magazines to the Library

Scientific journals, trade magazines, and business newspapers can show students a wide range of careers and help turn students on to the opportunities available after they graduate. Every profession, from the most complex to the practical, has its trade journal. Trade magazines are published in fields as diverse as banking, baking, car wash operation, construction, building maintenance, electronics, and many others. Parents who already work in these fields could bring their old trade journals to the school library. These magazines would provide a window into the world of jobs and help motivate students.

Additional Math, Science, and Graphics Resources

About.com's Animation Channel: Free animation software, plus free articles and tutorials. *animation.about.com*

Foldit: An online game where students can solve protein-folding chemistry problems and make real contributions to medical science.

Khan Academy: Free math and computer programming lessons. Learn JavaScript and other languages.

Code Academy: Free programming lessons

Udacity: Programming classes

Coursera: Online college courses

Type *Sketchup* into Google: Free drawing/3D-modeling software. *sketchup.google.com*

The National Science Digital Library: A national network of learning environments and resources for science, technology, engineering, and mathematics education at all levels. *nsdl.org*

OpenCourseWare Consortium: Free college course materials. *ocwconsortium.org*

Physics Education Technology (PhET): Fun, interactive, science simulations, from the PhET project at the University of Colorado. *phet.colorado. edu*

Wolfram Alpha: A knowledge engine that doesn't find information, but instead computes information based on built-in data, algorithms, and methods. *wolframalpha.com*

Wolfram MathWorld: A really awesome mathematics site that serves as a wiki encyclopedia of equations, theorems, algorithms, and more. *mathworld.wolfram.com*

If my third-grade teacher had continued trying to teach me to read with endless, boring drills, I would have failed the reading competency tests.

Getting Kids Turned On to Reading

O ne complaint I am hearing from both parents and teachers is that common core standards makes it impossible to spend much time on subjects other than reading and math because school districts put so much emphasis on students passing tests in these subjects. Recently, I had a discussion with a mom about teaching reading. She told me that her daughter, who has reading problems, was not allowed to go outside for recess because she had to do reading drills. The girl was bored stiff and hated it. However, she quickly learned to read when her mom taught her from a Harry Potter book. To motivate kids, especially those with autism spectrum disorders, you need to start with books the kids want to read. The Harry Potter series is one of the best things that has happened to reading instruction. Two hours before the last Harry Potter book went on sale, I visited the local Barnes and Noble. It was jammed full of kids in costume and a line stretched halfway around the block. I think it is wonderful that the kids were getting so turned on about a book.

I could not read when I was in third-grade. Mother taught me to read after school from an interesting book about Clara Barton, a famous nurse.

The content kept me interested, and motivated me to learn, even though the book was written at the sixth-grade level.

Mother taught me how to sound out the words, and within three months, my reading skills jumped two grade levels on standardized tests. I was a phonics learner, but other kids on the autism spectrum are visual, sight-word learners. When they read the word *dog*, they see a picture of a dog in their head. Children are different; parents should identify which way their child learns best and then use that method. There is now scientific evidence that there are separate neural pathways for either visually mapping whole words or decoding them phonologically.

Sight-word readers usually learn nouns first. To learn the meaning of words like *went* and *going* I had to see them in a sentence I could visualize. For example, "I *went* to the supermarket" or "I am *going* to the supermarket." One is past and the other is future. When I went to the supermarket I see myself with the bag of groceries I purchased. When I say I am *going* to the supermarket, I see myself driving there. Use examples the child can visualize and relate to when teaching all the connector words that are not easily visualized themselves.

If my third-grade teacher had continued trying to teach me to read with endless, boring drills, I would have failed the reading competency tests required by school systems that are "teaching to the test" to obtain better school-wide ranking on standardized tests. After Mother taught me reading, I was able to do really well on the elementary school reading tests. She got me engaged in reading in a way that was meaningful to me until reading became naturally reinforcing on its own.

Parents and teachers can use a child's special interests or natural talents in creative ways to teach basic academic skills such as reading and math. Science and history make wonderfully interesting topics to teach both subjects to spectrum children. If the child likes dinosaurs, teach reading using books about dinosaurs. A simple math problem might be rewritten using dinosaurs as the subject or new exercises created by the adult. For example: if a dinosaur walks at five miles per hour, how far can he walk in fifteen minutes?

Students with ASD can get excellent scores on standardized tests when more creative methods are used that appeal to their interests and ways of thinking. Although this creative effort may take a little more time at the onset, the improved learning, interest and motivation in the child will more than make up for the extra time in the long run.

Reference

Moseley, R.L. et al. (2014). Brain routes for reading in adults with and without autism: EMEG evidence. *J Autism Dev Disord.* 44:137-153.

Too Much Video Gaming and Screen Time has a Bad Effect on Child Development

A t conferences, more and more parents of a recently diagnosed teen or elementary school child have told me that they may be on the autism spectrum. In some cases, they have an official diagnoses and in other cases, they do not. Almost all the parents who have been told me that they are on the autism spectrum have worked successfully in a variety of occupations. The question is: why was their life relatively successful, and their child is having problems with lack of friends, bullying, or is extremely hyper and anxious? In most of these cases, the child has no early childhood speech delay. A possible contributor to a poorer prognosis may be excessive use of video games or other on-screen entertainment. When I was in college, I had friends who today would be labeled as having autism. Individuals on the autism spectrum are more likely to have pathological video game use. The ICD-11 now has a formal diagnosis for gaming disorder. Research shows that eight percent of all young people who play video games may be true addicts.

There may be two reasons why both these mildly autistic parents and my geeky classmates got and kept decent jobs.

1. They learned how to work at a young age. I have written extensively about this.

2. In my generation, kids played outside with their peers and learned social interactions. They were not glued to electronic screens.

In the September/October 2016 Carlat Report of Child Psychiatry, I read two articles that were a great "light bulb" moment. One was written by Mary G. Burke, M.D., psychiatrist at the Sutter Pacific Medical foundation in San Francisco, and the other was an interview with Michael Robb, PH.D. of Common Sense media. Dr. Burke explained that both babies and children need to engage with other people who react to their behavior. The problem with watching endless videos is that the video does not react to the child's responses. Today, Michael Robb recommends no more than 10 hours of screen time a week until the kids are in high school. This is the same rule my mother enforced for TV watching. The American Academy of Pediatrics recommends limited screen time to one to two hours a day. For young children under 18 months, the American Psychological Association recommends no screen time except for video chatting with people they know.

Electronic-Device-Free Times

Both specialists recommend that every family should have specific electronic-device-free times so they can interact and talk. There should be at least one device-free meal per day where both parents and children turn off and put all electronic devices away. In her practice, Dr. Burke has observed that reducing use of electronics reduces symptoms of OCD, panic attacks, and hyperactivity. According to The Centers of Disease Control, the diagnosis of ADHD or attention deficit has increased. Overuse of screens may be a contributor to this problem.

One study showed that a session of five days at an outdoor nature camp with no electronics improved the ability of middle school children to read non-verbal social cues. A farmer who ran a summer camp for eight- to eleven-year-olds had an interesting observation. During afternoon periods of free play in a walnut orchard, the boys sulked around for the first two days. On the third day, she told me, a switch flipped and they discovered free play. My three recommendations are:

1. Have one electronic-device-free meal where everybody—including parents—puts away all screens.
2. Limit video watching and video games, and other non-school screen time to 10 hours a week.
3. Engage the entire family in activities where people have to interact with each other.

Technology Industry Parents Restrict Electronics

The people who make electronic media in Silicon Valley are greatly restricting their children's use of video games and video watching. Two articles in the *New York Times* and *Business Insider* clearly show that the people who create the technology are concerned about their own children's use of electronics. Research is now showing that people on the autism spectrum are at a greater risk of developing video game addictions. When I talk to parents at autism meetings, I am observing two pathways for fully verbal young adults. The ones with the best outcomes learn how to hold a job before graduation from either high school or college. The ones with the poorest outcome may play video games for three to eight hours every day. Some of these kids have not been taught basic skills, such as shopping by themselves.

Friends Through Online Multi-Player Games

There are a number of papers that show that games where teens can talk to their friends can have some positive effects. Low to moderate use of multiplayer games would be one hour a day on weekdays and two hours a day on weekends. These games, when used in moderation, may help a child make and keep friends. When used properly with parental supervision, the online friendships can be turned into friendships in person. Children need to be taught to plan their play so that they do not have to stop in the middle of a Fortnite match. To do this, they may have to have no video games on one night in order to have sufficient time to complete a match on the next night. Some enterprising parents have developed activities to connect video games back to the real world. They went to the lumberyard and bought wood that was sanded and painted to create MineCraft blocks. One child with autism became the center of attention in his neighborhood with MineCraft blocks in his home's driveway.

There will be some situations where getting a child to disengage from a video game becomes so difficult that the games may have to be banned. A free paper is available online titled "Measuring DSM-5 Internet Gaming Disorder: Development Validation of a Short Psychometric Scale." It has nine questions to help determine if an individual has problem video game use. Some of the internet gaming disorder questions are:

1. Feeling more irritability, anxiety, or sadness when an attempt is made to reduce video game use.
2. Loss of interest in other hobbies or activities.
3. Jeopardizing jobs, education, or career.

How Can Video Games Be Harmful?

Video games can reduce empathy. Realistic killing of people or animals and showing cruelty and gore would be much more damaging than a game where inanimate objects or cartoon characters are destroyed. It is my opinion that images that enable a game player to graphically inflict pain and suffering on realistic human images are likely to be the most damaging. Douglas Gentle at Iowa State University reported that a meta-analysis of 136 scientific articles on violent video games showed that playing them led to desensitization and aggressive behavior (Bavelier et al., 2011). However, I believe that the nature of the violence is important. When I was a child, my hero was the Lone Ranger. He shot lots of bad guys who fell off their horses. In these shows, many people were shot, but they never showed realistic depictions of cruelty or suffering.

Pictures of car crashes or exploding aliens do not bother me. Violence done to objects, such as cars and buildings, does not have the same effect on me as graphic depictions of cruelty and torture. Since I am a visual thinker, I avoid movies that show graphic images of violence or cruelty. I do not want these pictures in my memory. In many movies, I analyze chase scenes and think, "This is impossible. A car cannot crash into a storefront and still be drivable." I am especially concerned when young children play realistic killings games. Little kids need to learn to control aggressive impulses. Canadian researchers have found that some children, especially in disadvantaged homes, show violent tendencies before age six that may lead to criminal behavior unless the child is taught how to control aggression. (Dr. Michael Rush at Boston's Children's Hospital can help you determine if your child spends too much time online (See Reddy, 2019).

In conclusion, video game use should be limited. I usually do not recommend banning it. A child needs to have enough experiences so he/she learns that there are many things in the world that are more interesting than video games.

References

Bavelier, D.C., Green, C.S., Han, D.H., Renshaw, P.F., Merzenich, M.M. and Gentile, D.A. (2011). Brains on video games, *Nature Review of Neuroscience* 12(12):763-768.

Bowles, N. (2018) A dark consensus about screens and kids begins to emerge in Silicon Valley, *New York Times*, October 26, 2018.

CDC (2016) Attention-Deficit/Hyperactivity Disorder (ADHD) Data and statistics cdc.gov (accessed June 28, 2019).

Courtwright, D.T. (2019) *The Age of Addiction: How Bad Habits Became Bug Business*, Harvard University Press.

Englehardt, C. and Mazurek, M.O. (2013) Video game access, parental rules and problem behavior: A study of boys with autism spectrum disorder, *Autism* (October). 18:529-587.

Englehardt, C. et al. (2017) Pathological game use in adults with and without autism spectrum disorder, *Peer Journal* 5:e3393.

Increasing prevalence of parent reported attention deficit/hyperactivity disorders among children, United States, 2003-2007.

Franklin, N., and Hunt, J. (2012) Rated E – Keeping up with our patient's video game playing, *The Brown University Child and Adolescent Behavior Letter* 28(3):1-5 doi: 10.1002/chi.20159.

Hall, S.S. (2014) The accidental epigenticist, *Science* 505:14-17.

Jargon, J. (2019) Gaming as a social bridge, *The Wall Street Journal*, June 26, 2019, pp. A13.

Kuss, D.J. et al. (2018) Neurobiological correlates in internet gaming disorder: A systematic literature review, *Frontiers in Psychiatry*, 9:166 10:3389/fpsyt.2018.00166.

Mazurek, M., Shattuck, P., Wagner, M., Cooper, B. December 8, 2011, Prevalence and correlates of screen-based media use among youths with autism spectrum disorders. *Journal of Autism and Development Disorders*. Available at: www.springerlink.comcontent/98412t131480547.

Mazurek, M.O., and Englehardt, C.R. (2013) Video games use in boys with autism spectrum disorder, ADHD or typical development, *Pediatrics* 132:260-266.

Mazurek, M.O. et al. (2015) Video games from the perspective of adults on the autism spectrum disorder, *Computers in Human Behavior*, 51:122-130.

Pontes, H.M. et al. (2015) Measuring DSM-5 internet gaming disorder: Development and validation of a short psychrometric scale. *Computers and Human Behavior*, 45:137-143 http://dx.doi,org/10.1016/j.chb.2014.12.006

Reddy, S. (2019) How to tell if your kids spend too much time online, *The Wall Street Journal*, p. A13, June 18, 2019.

Stone, B.G. et al. (2018) Online multiplayer games for social interactions of children with autism spectrum disorder: A resource for inclusive education, *International Journal of Inclusive Education*, pp. 1-20.

Sundburg, M. (2017) Online gaming loneliness and friendships among adolescents and adults with ASD, *Computers in Human Behavior*, https:doiorg/10.1016/j.chb.2017.10-020

Uhls, Y.T. et al. (2014) Five days at outdoor education camp without screens improves preteen skills with nonverbal emotion cues, *Computers and Human Behavior*, 39:387-392.

Welles, C. (2018) Silicon Valley parents are raising their kids tech free and it should be a red flag, BusinessInsider.com.

Therapy Animals and Autism

A s I travel around the country to talk with parents of individuals with ASD, more of them are asking whether they should get a service dog for their child with autism. The use of service or assistance dogs with spectrum children is gaining popularity, and there is increasing scientific evidence that service dogs are beneficial. However, this is a complicated issue. Unlike other autism interventions that can be more easily started and stopped, embarking on the journey to find an appropriate service dog for a child is a long-term commitment on the part of the entire family. A service dog is much more than a well-trained pet.

The first question I ask is, "Does your child like dogs?" If the family does not already own a dog, I suggest they see how their child will react to a friend's friendly dog first. There are three kinds of reactions the child can have. The first is an almost magical connection with dogs. The child and the dog are best buddies. They love being together. The second type of reaction is a child who may be initially hesitant but gets to really like dogs. The child should be carefully introduced to a calm, friendly dog. The third type of reaction is avoidance or fear. Often, the child who avoids dogs has a sensory issue. For instance, a child with sensitive hearing may be afraid of the dog's bark because it hurts his/her ears.

When I was a small child, the sound of the school bell hurt my ears like a dentist drill hitting a nerve. To a child with severe sound sensitivity, a dog may be perceived as a dangerous, unpredictable thing that can make a hurtful sound at any moment. For some individuals, the smell of a dog may be overpowering, although keeping the dog clean may alleviate this issue.

I also ask parents if they are willing and able to make the time, financial, and commotional commitment of having a service dog. This is a family affair, with everyone in the family involved. Waiting lists can be two years or more and fees for the trained dog can run $10,000 or more initially, and several thousand dollars each year thereafter.

Types of Service Dogs

There are three basic types of service dogs that are most likely to be used for individuals with autism. They are therapy dogs, a companion dog or a safety dog. A therapy dog is owned by a teacher or therapist and is used during lessons to facilitate learning. A companion dog lives with the family and spends most of its day interacting with the individual with autism. The dog can assist with social, emotional, behavioral, and sensory challenges in the child. These dogs also serve as a "social ice breaker" because other people are often attracted to a dog and will interact more readily with the child. Some individuals with autism really open up and interact with a dog.

Therapy dogs and companion service dogs must have basic obedience training plus training for public access. Companion service dogs usually receive additional training that focuses specifically on the needs of the child for whom it has been matched. For more information on training standards, visit the International Association of Assistance Dog Partners' website (iaadp.org).

The third type of service dog is the safety dog. These are highly trained service dogs used with individuals with severe autism who tend to run off. The child is tethered to the dog and the dog becomes a protector of sorts for the child. Safety dogs have to be used carefully to avoid stressing the dog. These animals need time off to play and just be a dog.

Dogs that are chosen to be assistance/service dogs should be calm, friendly, and show absolutely no signs of aggression toward strange people. They have to be trained for good manners in public such as not jumping on or sniffing people and not barking. This level of basic training is the absolute minimum any therapy or companion service dogs should obtain. Advanced training to become familiar with the behaviors of people with ASD is preferable.

Rules for Access to Public Places with Dogs

The Americans with Disabilities Act (ADA) has specific rules. A true service dog is allowed in ALL public places. An emotional support dog is not a service dog according to the ADA, but it does have more privileges than a regular dog. To be designated as a service dog, the animal is "trained to do work or perform a task for a person with a disability." It performs a task the person cannot do themselves. A service dog can also do a task such as detecting the start of a panic attack. To be designated as an emotional support animal, the person must have a diagnosis form a doctor or mental health professional. Emotional support animals (ESA) are allowed on airlines. People must act responsibly when it comes to their dogs traveling with them. If they continue to act as irresponsible pet owners, ESA animals could be kicked off the airlines. In one horrible case on Delta airlines, an ESA dog ripped up the face of another passenger. Please do not bring dogs that may bite into public areas unless they are muzzled.

There are many different groups who train companion and service dogs. One of the best ways to find a respectable source is through referrals from satisfied people who have service dogs. It is also important to train the dog to know the difference between work and play behavior. A dog's brain will create categories of behavior. When the vest is on, he works, and when the vest is off, it's time to play. The dog needs to be taught clear "vest on" and "vest off" behavior.

Questions to Ask when Selecting a Service Dog Provider

- What breeds of dogs do you use for autism assistance dogs?
- Can we (the family) assist in selecting the dog for our child?
- Do you start the process with puppies, or are your placements fully grown dogs?
- If puppies, what will happen if my child doesn't take to the dog? What if the dog's maturing personality becomes mismatched to my child?
- If an adult dog (two years or older), has the dog been trained specifically with ASD behaviors in mind, or has training been generalized to people with other disabilities instead?
- Describe the training program the dog receives. How long does it last and to what extent is our family involved?
- Does the training address socialization issues only, or are the dogs trained to handle run away situations, sensory sensitivities, behavioral challenges, emergency situations, etc.?
- Will the dog be trained with my child's specific needs/behaviors in mind?
- At what age will the dog come into our home?
- Has/will the dog be trained to respond to hand signals in addition to verbal commands? This is especially important if the child is nonverbal or has limited verbal skills.
- How many dog placements with children with autism has your organization completed?

- How successful were these placements over time?
- How much family training with the dog is required/provided to us? Does this include training with the spectrum child, or just with parents?
- Is there any "refresher" training provided at a future date?
- What type of ongoing communication with our family will be included once the dog is placed?
- Do you have references of families of children with ASD who own one of your dogs?
- What is your application procedure?
- Is there a wait list, and if so, how long?
- What are your fees for an assistance dog? Is there any financial assistance available for this? Do you provide a payment plan over time?
- What type of expenses will our family incur over time in keeping the dog?
- There are lots of scams and fake service dog credentials. Be sure you are dealing with reputable people.

Therapy Dogs and Horses

There is increasing evidence that dogs, horses, and other animals can have definite therapeutic benefits. Animals that are used in therapy are often not trained service animals. For individuals with autism, dogs and horses can be really helpful in teaching social skills. The paper by Wijkeset (2019) has an extensive literature review.

Therapeutic riding is also becoming increasingly popular. When I was a teenager, my social life revolved around horses and I learned work skills by cleaning stalls. Many studies, including randomized trials show social benefits for individuals with autism. Real horse activities were much more effective than using a fake horse and barn activities with no horses present. I have observed many therapeutic riding programs. Sometimes there is a tendency to over accommodate a rider. I have observed many riders who still have a side walker who were capable of independent riding.

References and Additional Reading

Becker, J. and Rogers, E.C. (2017) Animal assisted social skills training for children with autism spectrum disorder, *Anthrozoos*, 302:307-326.

Berry, A. et al. (2013) Use of assistance and therapy dogs of children with autism spectrum disorders, *Journal of Alternative and Complimentary Medicine* 18:1-8.

Borgi, M. et al. (2016) Effectiveness of standardized equine assisted therapy program for children with autism spectrum disorder, *Journal of Autism and Developmental Disorder*, 46:1-9.

Brannon, S. et al. (2019) Service animals and emotional support animals where they are allowed and under what condition? ADA National Network, Information Guidance and Training in the American with Disabilities Act.

Burrows, K.E., Adams, C.L. and Millman, S.T. (2008) Factors affecting behavior and welfare of service dogs for children with autism spectrum disorder, *Journal of Applied Animal Welfare Science*, 11:42-62.

Burrows, K.E., Adams, C.L. and Spiers, J. (2008) Sentinels of safety: Service dogs ensure safety and enhance freedom and well-being for families with autistic children, *Quality Health Research*, 18:1642-1649.

Gabnals, R.L. et al. (2015) Randomized controlled trial of therapeutic horseback riding in children and adolescents with autism spectrum disorder, *American Academy of Child and Adolescent Psychiatry*, 54:541-549.

Grandin, T. (2011) The roles animals can play with individuals with autism, In: Peggy McCardle et al. (editors) *Animals in Our Lives*, Brookes Publishing, Baltimore, MD.

Grandin, T (2019) Case Study: How horses helped a teenager with autism make friends and learn how to work, *International Journal of Environmental Research and Public Health*, 16(13) 2325, doi.org/10.3390/jerph16132325.

Grandin, T., Fine, A.H. and Bowers, C.M. (2010) The use of therapy animals with individuals with autism, Third Edition, Therapeutic Foundations and Guidelines for Practice, A.H. Fine (Editor) *Animal Assisted Therapy*, Academic Press, San Diego, CA, 247-264.

Gross, P.D. (2005) *The Golden Bridge: A Guide to Assistance Dogs for Children Challenged by Autism and Other Developmental Disorders*, Purdue University Press, West Lafayette, IN.

Harris, A. et al. (2017) The impact of horse riding intervention on the social functioning of children with autism spectrum disorder, International *Journal of Environmental Public Health*, 14:776.

Llambias, C. et al. (2016) Equine assisted occupational therapy: Increasing engagement in children with autism spectrum disorder, *American Journal of Occupational Therapy*, 70, doi:10.5014/ajot.2016.02070.

O'Hare, M.E. (2013) Animal assisted intervention and autism spectrum disorders: A systematic literature review, *Journal of Autism and Developmental Disorders*, 43:1602-1622.

O'Hare, M.E. (2017) Research on animal assisted intervention and autism spectrum disorder, *Applied Developmental Science*, 21:200-215.

Pavlides, M. (2008) *Animal Assisted Interactions*, Jessica Kingsley Publishers, London, England.

Srinivasan, S.M. et al. (2018) Effects of equine therapy on individuals with autism spectrum disorder: A systematic review, *Review Journal of Autism Developmental Disorders*, 5:156-158.

Viau, R. et al. (2010) Effects of service dogs on salivary cortisol secretion in autistic children, *Psychoneuroendrocrinology*, 35:1187-1193.

Wijkes, C. et al. (2019) Effects of dog assisted therapy for adults with autism spectrum disorders: An exploratory randomized controlled trial, *Developmental Disorders*, doi.org/10.007/s10803-01903971-9.

Further Information

Autism Service Dogs of America
Autismservicedogsofamerica.com

Therapy Dogs International
www.tdi-dog.org

4 Paws 4 Ability,
4pawsforability.org/autismdogs.html

Paws Giving Independence
www.givingindependence.org

NEADS World Class Service Dogs
Neads.org

Assistance Dogs for Autism
Autismassistancedog.com

Pawsitivity Service Dogs
Pawsitivityservicedogs.com

The Importance of Choices

S ometimes it is difficult to get children and teens on the spectrum to do new things or participate in everyday activities. When I was afraid to go to my aunt's ranch, Mother gave me the choice of going for either two weeks or all summer. Giving me a choice helped prevent the problem of the option to say "no." Individuals on the spectrum often do better when they have some options or control over their environment. Many parents have told me that their child will often say "no" and refuse to do something. Allowing the child to have some choices will help prevent a lot of stubbornness or oppositional behavior. When there is a choice, it is difficult for the child to answer with "no."

The Right School for Me

My mother allowed me to have choices about how I was going to participate in a new situation. After I was kicked out of a large girl's school because I retaliated for teasing by throwing a book at another girl, my mother had to find a new school for me. Fortunately, she had worked as a TV journalist on two documentaries, so she had already visited many specialized schools in a three-state area near where we lived. First, she narrowed down the list of possibilities by choosing three schools she had visited that she really liked. I had the chance to visit all three schools. I had extensive tours so I could find out what the schools were really like. Then, mother allowed me to pick one of the three schools.

Limiting Access to Video Games

For some children, it will be essential to limit their time spent on video games. One good way to do this is by establishing the length of time a video game can be accessed and then allowing the child to decide when he will use the allotted time to do so. A child could be given a choice of playing the game for one hour when he returns home from school. This could be effective in helping him calm down from a long day at school. Or, the child could choose to play the game for one hour after homework is done. No matter which choice the child makes, he is still playing for only one hour.

Personalizing Personal Hygiene

There is a scene in the movie *Temple Grandin* where my boss slams down a deodorant stick and says, "You stink; use it." This actually happened! Hygiene is often a major issue with teenagers on the spectrum. One way this can be approached is to give the teen some choices of hygiene products to use. What is nonnegotiable is that the teen will have to take a bath or shower every day. However, he can go to the store and choose the soaps or products he will use.

In the past, the selection of hygiene products was limited. I hated the gooey sticky roll-on deodorants that were common in the 1970s. Today there is a wide assortment of products to choose from. (I like the solid, unscented deodorant stick the best.) Scent can also be a big issue in the hygiene product department: it's important that the scent is not overpowering to the individual, or the product is less likely to be used!

Acquisition of Daily Living Skills

There are lots of skills that kids have to learn (e.g., getting dressed, table manners, and household chores). Getting the child to comply is often easier if choices are provided in conjunction with the daily living skills.

Getting dressed. Often getting ready in the morning can be a struggle for young kids on the spectrum. It can be as simple as allowing the child a choice between two different shirts. I chose my clothes and laid them out the night before.

Table manners. At the dinner table, mother insisted on good manners. At the end of the meal, I had a choice. I could ask to be excused early with no dessert or wait and get dessert. Those were the two choices. Leaving early and getting dessert was not allowed.

Household chores. When children feel like they have some say in things, they are much more likely to want to learn and practice skills such as cleaning, picking up toys, and loading the dishwasher. If three chores need to be completed before a child has free time, you could let the child choose the order the chores will be completed in.

It is important to give children choices because many individuals have a reflex reaction to say "no." Letting the child have choices will give his mind time to stop and think instead of going into a reflexive "no" mode. Finesse the "no" with choices, and everyday life can flow much more smoothly for parent and child.

Remember a basic principle in working with autistic individuals: an obsession or fixation has huge motivational potential for the child.

The Importance of Practical Problem-Solving Skills

Both normal children and kids on the autism spectrum need to be challenged. Those who have heard me speak or read my books know I think many parents and educators coddle their children with ASD far more than they should. Children with ASD don't belong in a bubble, sheltered from the normal experiences of the world around them. Sensory issues do need to be taken into consideration, but aside from those, parents may need to push their child a little for any real advancement in learning to occur.

This is especially true in teaching a pivotal life skill: problem-solving. It involves training the brain to be organized, break down tasks into step-by-step sequences, relate parts to the whole, stay on task, and experience a sense of personal accomplishment once the problem is solved. Young kids learn by doing, and kids with ASD often learn best with concrete, visible examples. When I was a child growing up in the '50s, I built tree houses and went on backyard campouts with other neighborhood children. In those situations, several children had to work together to figure out how to ac-complish the task. We had to find lumber for the tree house, design it, take measurements, and discuss how to get the boards up the tree and nailed into place. We learned by trying different things; some things worked, others did not. Experiments with wetting lumber to make it easier to cut with a hand saw were a complete failure.

From our experiences, we learned that dry lumber was easier to cut. The rigorous turn-taking training I had when I was 3-6 years old served me well in these group activities. In our family we played lots of board games—an excellent teaching method for learning how to take turns. Turn-taking helped me understand that people can work together for a common purpose, that what one person did could affect me and the outcome of the game positively or negatively. It made me aware of different perspectives, which in turn helped me become a better detective when I had to solve a problem.

I can remember the huge planning meetings we had for the backyard campout. There was candy and soda that had to be bought. We all had to figure out how to put up an old army tent. None of the parents helped, which made it a valuable learning experience for us all.

Like myself, many kids with ASD have a natural curiosity about certain things. These interests can be used constructively to practice problem-solving skills. I loved toys that flew. On a windy day, a parachute I made from a scarf would fly for hundreds of feet. But not on the first try. It took many attempts before I was successful. I had to figure out how to prevent the strings from tangling when I threw the parachute up into the air. I tried building a cross from two pieces of 5" coat-hanger wire to tie the four strings to; it worked. When I was in high school, I was fascinated with optical illusions. After seeing an illusion called the Ames Trapezoidal Window, I wanted to build one. My science teacher challenged me to try to figure it out by myself rather than giving me a book with a diagram. I spent six months working on it, without success. Then my teacher let me have a brief glimpse at a photo in a textbook that showed how the illusion worked. He gave me a hint without telling me exactly how to do it. He helped me develop problem-solving skills.

Children with ASD (and many of their parents) struggle with problem-solving skills today. This may be partially due to us,

as a society, doing less hands-on practical work and activities than did our counterparts when I was growing up. We fix less; we toss things out that don't work and buy new ones. Even in today's internet world, there is a need for problem-solving skills. The key is to start with concrete, hands-on projects that have meaning for the child, then slowly move into abstract problem solving involving thoughts and creativity, in academics and social situations. The ability to solve problems helps a person categorize and use the vast amounts of information in his mind, and from outside sources like the internet, in a successful, intelligent manner. These are important life-skills and parents should start early in incorporating problem-solving opportunities into their child's daily routine.

The ability to produce work that pleases others is an essential skill for successful employment.

Learning to Do Assignments That Other People Appreciate

R ecently I was looking through my old high school album. As I looked through my old photos, I realized I had learned an important skill by the time I was in high school that some people on the autism spectrum never learn. I had photo after photo of projects I had created that pleased others. There was a gate I had built for my aunt out at the ranch and sets I had made for the school play. There were also before and after pictures of the ski tow house I refurbished at my boarding school. Originally we had a homemade rope tow in an ugly, plywood shed. I put tongue and groove wood siding on the ski tow house, stained it, and then installed white trim around the windows and door. It was decorated the way others would like it. Left to my own preferences, I would have painted pictures of goofy cartoons on it, but that would not have earned the approval of my teachers. In all three projects, I created things taking into consideration the thoughts and preferences of others in my environment. The end result was positive recognition for my work.

During my elementary school years, my mother, my nanny, and my teachers taught me—first in direct and later in indirect ways—that sometimes you can do things to please just yourself, but other times you need to do things that others would like. They also made sure I understood that sometimes this was a choice, while at other times it was mandatory. This is an important and pivotal life skill, and it's an advantage if you can learn it early in childhood. It affects whether or not a child is accepted by his or her peer group, and how well he can work with others. Even as a young child I did projects that pleased others. When I was in fourth grade, I sewed costumes for the school play with my little toy sewing machine. I quickly learned in school that, in order to get good grades, I needed to attend to my teachers' requests, and follow directions. It did no good to turn in a brilliant report if I hadn't addressed the assignment.

Both as a young child and throughout my high school years I was motivated by two factors. The first was getting recognition from others and, secondly, I enjoyed seeing my creations being used in places and events that were important to me.

As children grow into young adults, the ability to produce work that pleases others is an *essential* skill for successful employment. Students on the spectrum should be taught these essential skills well before they graduate from high school. The teaching should start early, while the child is young, in concrete ways. Educators and parents must teach these individuals to successfully complete assignments that fit somebody else's specifications. If a student is in a robotics club, he has to learn to make a robot that will do an *assigned* task. A student in middle school English class must learn to write an essay that addresses the specific question posed, even when it's not something interesting to him.

Recently I met a bright man with Asperger's Syndrome who had just graduated from college. He had absolutely no work experience while he was in high school and college, and absolutely no idea of how to get and keep a job. He had never mowed somebody else's lawn or worked in a store. Other than academics, he had never been put into situations where he needed to satisfactorily produce work according to someone else's directions. By the time I graduated from college I had already done many jobs and internships. Mother realized that preparing me for the world outside my home needed to start slowly and easily, and build, one event, one project, one skill upon another.

Teachers, parents, and therapists must help high-functioning students on the spectrum learn how to do projects to another person's specification. I did not realize how well I had learned this skill until I looked at my old high school photos. This hindsight helped me further realize how much I have grown and developed since then.

Learning is a constant process for us all. However, the child with autism relies on his parents and teachers to look forward at the life skills necessary for survival and success, and begin teaching these skills early in life.

It is never too late to expand the mind of a person on the autism spectrum.

Learning Never Stops

After I turned 50, many people told me my talks kept getting better and smoother. One thing many people do not realize about people on the autism spectrum is that they never stop growing and developing. Each day I learn more and more about how to behave and communicate.

Autistic thought is bottom-up thinking instead of top down, as it is in most people. To form a concept, I put lots of little pieces of information together. The normal person forms a concept first and then attempts to make all the details fit. The older I get the more data I collect and the better I become at forming concepts. Being exposed to many new experiences has helped me load more information into the database in my mind, my memory. I have more and more information to help me know how to deal with new situations. To understand something new, I have to compare it to something I have already experienced.

Internet in My Head

The best analogy to how my mind works is this: it is like having an internet inside my head. The only way my internal internet can get information is through reading or actual experiences. My mind also has a search engine that works like Google for pictures. When somebody says a word, I see pictures in my imagination. I have to have visual images to think. When

I was younger, the library of pictures in my head was much smaller, so I had to use visual symbols to understand new concepts. In high school, I used door symbols to represent thinking about my future. To think about my future after high school, I practiced walking through an actual door that symbolized my future. Without the door symbol, my future was too abstract for me to understand.

Today I no longer use door symbols because they have been replaced with pictures of other things I have experienced or things I have read. When I read a book with descriptive text, I translate it into photorealistic pictures. As more and more different things are experienced, the more flexible my thinking becomes because the "photo internet" in my head has more pictures and information to surf through.

Exposure to New Things is Essential

Exposing children and adults on the autism/Asperger's spectrum to new things is really important. Mother was always making me try new things, and some I did not like, but I still did them. When I was about twelve years old, Mother enrolled me in a children's sail boating program, two afternoons a week, all summer. It was a poorly run program and I hated it after the first few sessions because I had no buddy to do it with, yet I completed all the sessions. The lesson I learned was that if you start something, you have to finish it.

As an adult I motivate myself to keep learning through extensive reading and personal/professional experiences. In the last ten years of my life, from my fifties to my sixties, I have still improved. One revelation I had around age fifty was learning that humans use little eye signals that I did not know existed. I learned about eye signals from the book, *Mind Blindness* by Simon Baron-Cohen. When I read autism literature I gain great insight from both personal accounts of people on the autism spectrum and neuroscience research. Scientific research has helped me understand how my brain is different. That has helped me comprehend "normal" people better.

Doing Assignments

A few years ago I realized the extent to which the training I had in my childhood and teens really helped me later in life. High school was torture with the incessant teasing and I was a goof-off student with little interest in studying. For years I have written about how my science teacher motivated me to study so I could become a scientist. His mentoring was extremely important. Lately I have realized that although I was not studying in school, I had very good work skills that helped me later in the world of employment. I did lots of work that other people appreciated. I cleaned the horse stalls, shingled the barn roof, and painted signs. Even though I got obsessed with these activities, it was useful work that other people wanted done.

To be successful, people on the spectrum have to learn how to take their skills and do an assignment. The ability to do an assignment (follow directions, stay on task, complete it in a satisfactory manner) was taught to me from a young age. In grade school, my ability in art was encouraged but I was repeatedly asked to create pictures of many different things (again, producing work for others). I enjoyed the praise I got when I drew a picture of something somebody else had requested.

Parents and teachers can lay the groundwork for a child's later success in life by exposing the child to many new experiences. But children and adults of all ages can continue to grow and evolve in their behavior and thinking. It is never too late to expand the mind of a person on the autism spectrum.

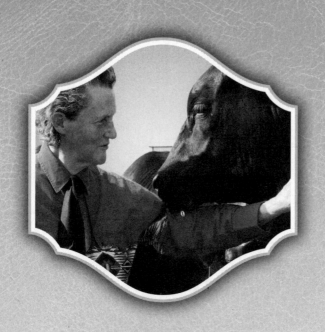

CHAPTER 3

Sensory Issues

One of the problems in understanding sensory issues is that sensory sensitivities are very variable, among individuals and within the same individual.

I have been talking and writing about sensory problems for over thirty years and I am still perplexed by many people who do not acknowledge sensory issues and the pain and discomfort they can cause. A person doesn't have to be on the autism spectrum to be affected by sensory issues. In fact, a study at Cardiff University showed that mothers of children with autism often have atypical sensory reactions. Most people feel an aversion to nails being drawn across a chalkboard. That's a negative sensory experience. Many times I have heard of people who get almost instant headaches when exposed to certain scents, like strong perfumes or the smell of gasoline. That's a sensory experience. A woman I know tells me her hearing is very sensitive when she first wakes up in the morning, and even normal sounds are sometimes offensive for the first thirty minutes or so. That's a sensory challenge. Think about going to the mall and shopping on a busy Saturday afternoon. For some it's energizing, but for others, it leaves them exhausted. These people are having trouble with the sensory bombardments that are typical of the mall environment: the constantly changing sights, smells, voices, music, and being bumped into by others, etc. Sensory issues are very real, and I think they are more a matter of degree than being either present or absent in people. I also believe that as our world in general gets louder and busier with more people, more cars, more urbanization, and a heavier reliance on technology, sensory issues will become more pervasive as our sensory systems become increasingly overloaded.

For me and other people on the autism spectrum, sensory experiences that have little or no effect on neurotypical people can be severe life stressors for us. Loud noises hurt my ears like a dentist's drill hitting a nerve. For some individuals, the seams in a pair of socks or the rough texture of materials like wool can feel like being constantly burned. This explains why a child's reaction is to take them off—he's not being defiant; the socks are physically hurting him. For others, even the light touch of another's hand on their arm can be painful. They shrink away from people not because they are antisocial, but because even brushing up against another person can feel like razors drawn across their skin.

I think so many professionals and nonprofessionals have ignored sensory issues because they just can't imagine that an alternate sensory reality exists if they have not experienced it personally. They simply cannot imagine it, so it does not register in their minds. That type of narrow perception, however, does nothing to help individuals who do have these very real issues in their lives. Even if they don't understand it on a personal level, it's time they put aside their personal ideas. Scientific research has now documented that sensory problems are real. Higher functioning adults with autism and Asperger's are writing about their sensory issues in great detail. Many of these individuals agree that sensory issues are the primary challenge of autism in their daily lives. There is a great need for more scientific research on the brain abnormalities that are associated with different sensory problems and methods to treat them.

Sensory Problems Are Variable

O ne of the problems in understanding sensory issues is that sensory sensitivities are very variable, among individuals and within the same individual. A person can be hyper-sensitive in one area (like hearing) and hypo-sensitive in another (like touch). One person can have a marked olfactory sensitivity and another might not be affected at all in that sense. Complicating matters even further, on a day-to-day basis, in the same individual, the sensory sensitivities can change, especially when the person is tired or stressed. These many and constantly shifting variables make it difficult to design research studies to test therapies to treat sensory sensitivities. So professionals will loudly make assertions such as "There is no research to support sensory integration therapy with individuals with autism"—tacitly suggesting the therapy is ineffective.

The absence of clinical research does not mean sensory therapies are not viable for children or adults. It simply means research has not been done to date. Furthermore, with the variable nature of sensory issues in autism, we must look at research with a slightly different slant. If twenty children are put in a study and four benefit from the therapy, while sixteen don't, is it ethical to deem the therapy ineffective? It really worked on four children. Four children's lives are now markedly different; their world is no longer hellish to live in. A better approach in situations like this is to delve deeper into why it works for some, and not for others, to continue to explore what is going on in their brains by doing follow-up research between the responders and non-responders, rather than arbitrarily dismissing the therapy altogether.

There are two ways a child can respond to sensory overload: withdraw and shut off the world or scream and yell. Some children who appear to be non-responsive are actually in sensory shutdown due to sensory overload.

Parents and teachers often ask—"How can I tell if my child has sensory problems?" My simple answer is this: watch your child closely—the signs are there. Do you see him putting his hands over his ears to block out noise? Does he become agitated every time you're in a bustling, noisy, or chaotic environment? Are there certain textures of food he just will not tolerate? Do you find her pulling at or taking off clothes that have rough textures or tugging at necklines where tags are rubbing? Children and adults who tantrum and cannot tolerate being in a large supermarket, such as Wal-Mart, are almost certain to have sensory problems. Also note: tolerance levels quickly diminish when the individual is tired or hungry. For example, a child may tolerate a large grocery store in the morning but not during the afternoon.

Desensitization to Sensory Stimuli

Some children can learn to tolerate loud noises that they previously could not tolerate if they initiate the sound and have control of it. Let the child turn on the smoke alarm or other feared sound. Start with the volume low and gradually increase it. With the smoke alarm, you could start with it wrapped in heavy towels to muffle the sound and then gradually take them off. There MUST NEVER be a sudden surprise. The child must have control.

Easy Strategies

There are some simple things parents, educators, and service providers can do to help prevent sensory problems from hindering your child's education and life. Avoid multi-tasking, especially when working with the child. Have a quiet place free from outside distractions to do teaching, discrete trials, or other therapies. I have difficulty hearing if there is too much background noise— I can't discern my communication partner's voice from all the other sounds going on around me. Make sure the child gets lots of exercise every day. A significant number of research studies support the benefits of regular daily exercise. Exercise is really good for the brain and can help children with hyper-sensitivities calm down, and children with hypo-sensitivities rev up their system for optimal learning states. One of the articles in this section discusses simple ways to incorporate calming sensory activities into an educational program.

Sometimes very simple interventions can have amazing effects, as is described in the article on visual processing problems. The chapter on environmental enrichment provides more easily implemented strategies. For children who refuse to wear shoes, deep pressure massage of the feet immediately before putting on the shoes is sometimes helpful. One little girl could not tolerate a large supermarket for more than five minutes.

After her mother bought her a pair of children's pink-tinted sunglasses, she was able to get through an hour of shopping. Other children learn better when they are shielded from the distracting flicker of fluorescent lights. Some of the energy-saver fluorescent light bulbs have such a high degree of flicker that I cannot read with them. Some fluorescent lamps have electronic circuits to reduce flicker, but others make some people on the autism spectrum feel as though they are standing in the middle of a disco nightclub. (Try concentrating on a test in that type of environment! If fluorescent lights can't be avoided, a lamp with an old fashioned incandescent light bulb should be placed next to the child's desk to help eliminate flickers, or kids can wear baseball caps with longer brims to mask off some of the flicker. Switching to LED lamps may also be helpful.

Unfortunately, some LED lamps may also flicker. There are many new lamps that are becoming available. A visit to a lighting store where different lamps can be tried may help find lamps that do not flicker. At our university, students who had problems with seeing flickers visited many buildings on campus to discover which lamps did not flicker. They then purchased these lamps for their study and lounge areas.

Auditory Problems

Auditory challenges are often cited as the #1 sensory challenge among individuals with autism/Asperger's. There are two kinds of auditory problems: 1) sensitivity to loud noise in general and 2) not being able to hear auditory detail, such as discerning one voice among other sounds, or hearing the hard consonant sounds of words. An auditory sensitivity to noises, where sounds hurt the ears, can be extremely debilitating. Sound sensitivity can make it impossible for some people on the spectrum to tolerate normal places such as restaurants, offices, and sports events. These extreme auditory problems can occur in both nonverbal individuals and those who are very high-functioning with marked intelligence and language capabilities, such as college educated people with Asperger's.

Auditory training therapy is useful for some people. In auditory training, a person listens to electronically distorted music a couple of sessions a day for ten days. The music sounds like an old-fashioned record player that is speeding up and slowing down. AT helps some children and adults, yet has no effect on others. The main improvements seen in those that it helps include reducing sound sensitivity and increasing hearing of auditory detail. For many children, getting their auditory input under control results in improved concentration and fewer behavior issues, giving other therapies and learning situations a chance to take hold. Some people with more minor auditory challenges use earplugs or music headphones to block out distracting or painful sounds, things such as chairs scraping on the floor in the cafeteria, the constant ringing of telephones in a busy office, or maneuvering through a crowded airport. Earplugs must never be worn all the time; this can cause the individual to become even more sensitive to sound. They need to be off at least half of the day, but can be used in noisy places such as shopping malls or the gym.

An Integrated Approach to Treatment

Severe sensory sensitivity can be a MAJOR barrier to learning in children, and in employment and socializing as the child grows and becomes an adult. My own sensory problems are minor nuisances, but for others, they can literally wreck the person's life. There are many highly intelligent adults with ASD or Asperger's, with brilliant minds in their field, who have such severe sensory issues that they cannot tolerate a normal job environment. They must either find ways to work independently from home, where they can control sensory input, or remain largely unemployed.

Employers are beginning to understand sensory issues and some will even make accommodations when the needs of the person are explained. However, on the whole, we as a society have far to go in appreciating the challenge of living with sensory issues that most people on the autism spectrum face daily.

Teachers and parents should look closely for sensory issues in a child or young adult. Recurring behavior problems often have a sensory issue as the root cause of the behavior. If a sensory issue is suspected, a consultation with a good Occupational Therapist should be the next step. These individuals are trained to recognize sensory issues and then develop a customized program for the child. Interventions such as deep pressure, slow swinging, and games involving balancing work best when they are done every day.

Sensory issues are daily issues. If the services of an OT are available for only half an hour each week, parents and teachers should visit the session and ask the OT to show them what to do the rest of the week. For children, a combination of sensory therapies such as sensory integration from an OT, auditory training, and visual interventions coupled with other treatments works best. Special diets help some children with their sensory issues; improvements are seen not just in tolerating different textures and types of food, but also in other sensory areas as well. With older children and adults, a little dose of a conventional medication may reduce sound sensitivity if less invasive methods have proven unsuccessful.

Both Autism and ADHD Have Working Memory Problems

There is a lot of crossover between ASD and ADHD. I have talked to many parents whose child's diagnosis has been switched back and forth between autism and ADHD. Dr. Tara Stevens and her colleagues at Texas Tech University found that 59% of children who were diagnosed with ASD also had ADHD. This was more likely to occur in fully verbal children diagnosed after age six. Canadian researchers have also found that there were similarities in brain circuitry problems in both ASD and ADHD. Individuals with both labels are also more likely to have problems with working memory.

Give Them a Checklist

When I worked milking cows, I was saved by a checklist taped to the wall that outlined the steps on how to set up the equipment for milking and how to put it through the wash cycle afterward. The checklist helped me because I absolutely cannot remember a sequence of instructions. Set up required seven or eight steps, and wash up was another three or four. A checklist can help an individual on the spectrum keep their job. It will help prevent an employer from becoming frustrated when the person cannot remember how to operate a piece of equipment after being shown several times how to do it. For example, if a person with ASD gets at job at McDonald's, they will need a checklist to help them to remember the sequence for tearing down and cleaning the ice cream machine. After they have done it for a few weeks, they will have the process videotaped into their memory. At this point, the checklist may no longer be needed.

When I first started working in the meat-packing industry, I learned to remember the sequence of how the plant operated by videotaping the entire production line into my memory. This required many days of observation. Playing the "videotape" back in my imagination puts absolutely no load on working memory. In my imagination, I turn on the "video player" and walk through the plant. This videotape provides the sequence.

In conclusion, avoid giving long strings of verbal instruction. Demonstrate the task that requires a sequence of steps and provide a written checklist. Each bullet point on the checklist needs only three to five words to jog the memory.

Additional Reading

Ameis, S.H. et al. (2016. A diffusion tensor imaging study in children with ADHD, autism spectrum disorder, OCD, and matched controls, *American Journal of Psychiatry* (In press).

Ayres, J.A. 1979. *Sensory Integration and the Child.* Los Angeles, CA: Western Psychological Press.

Ben-Sasson, A., et al. 2009. A meta-analysis of sensory modu- lation symptoms in individuals with autism spectrum disorders. *Journal of Autism and Developmental Disorders* 39:1-11.

Blackmore, S.J. et al. 2006. Tactile sensitivity in Asperger syndrome. *Brain and Cognition* 61: 5-13.

Englund, J.A. et al. (2013) Common cognitive deficits in children with Attention Deficit Hyperactivity Disorder and Autism, *Journal of Psychoeducational Assessment*, Vol. 32, pp. 96-106.

Kercode, S. et al. (2014) Working memory and autism, *Research in Autism Spectrum Disorders*, Vol. 8, pp. 1316-1332.

A child who can see his world clearly has a much better chance of benefiting from other therapies.

Visual Processing Problems in Autism

Visual processing problems are common in individuals with autism spectrum disorder (ASD). They can result in lack of eye contact, staring at objects, or using side vision. These individuals may have difficulty with visually "holding still"; they constantly scan their surroundings for visual information in an attempt to gain meaning.

Suspect a visual processing problem if you see a child with ASD tilt his head and look out of the corner of his eye. Children or adults with visual processing difficulties can see flicker in 50or 60-cycle fluorescent lights, and they may have difficulty going up and down a strange set of stairs due to distorted depth perception. Most neurotypical children love to play on escalators, but a child with poor vision processing may fear the escalator. Some children and adults may have difficulty reading because black print on a white page will jiggle and vibrate. Adults with mild vision processing problems may hate driving at night.

Donna Williams, a well-known high functioning person with ASD, described her visual processing problems. Faces appeared like two-dimensional Picasso-like mosaics. High-contrasting colors in room décor were distressing. (In severe cases, it may be like the image on a flat-screen TV pixelating and breaking up.) Other individuals have complained that yellow and black caution stripes appear to vibrate. Motor, cognitive, speech, and perceptual abilities can all be affected when visual processing is impaired. Visual processing problems range from mild annoyances to very severe. These problems will not be evident in a regular eye exam because the malfunction is in the visual cortex.

Donna Williams and others have been helped by wearing pale tinted glasses. Tinted glasses have enabled some children and adults to tolerate a large store that is lighted with fluorescent lights. It is essential that the person is allowed to choose the color that works best for him. Stores that sell sunglasses have a wide variety of pale tinted glasses that may help reduce visual distortion, make reading easier, and increase the ability to tolerate 50- and 60-cycle fluorescent lights and highly contrasting room décor. Usually the light pink, lavender, gray, blue, or tan tints work best. The tints must be pale if the glasses are used for reading. Experiment by taking a book into a store with fluorescent lights and try reading with different tints.

Another aid that may be helpful is printing reading materials on tan, gray, or pastel paper to reduce contrast. Try a sample of every pale-colored paper at a local copy shop. The best paper color is often different from the best lens color.

The recommended computer screens to avoid flicker are laptops, tablets, and smartphones. You can also experiment with different colored backgrounds, type size, and fonts. There are some people who love their Kindle e-reader, which has a slightly gray background.

These are simple interventions that parents and teachers can experiment with at little or no cost. I have observed that these are most likely to work for the subset of individuals who answer yes to three screening questions: (1) Do you see the print jiggle on the page? (2) Do fluorescent lights bother you? and (3) Do you hate escalators because you have difficulty judging how to get on and off?

Scientific research on the use of colored lenses and colored overlays is full of conflicting results. Researchers who study migraine headaches and strokes report that colored filters improved reading (Beasley and Davis 2013; Huang et al. 2011). Other studies also indicated that colored filters were helpful for children diagnosed with ASD (Kaplan, Edelson, and Seip 1998; Ludlow, Taylor-Wiffen, and Wilkins 2012). However, research conducted with dyslexic college students (Henderson, Tsogka, and Snowling 2012) and school children (Ritchie, Sala, and McIntosh 2011) diagnosed with both Irlen syndrome and reading problems had no significant differences. The paper on Irlen syndrome has an extensive rebuttal in the comment section (Ritchie, Sala, and McIntosh 2011). British researchers found that colored filters help control cortical hyperexcitability.

Today with all the emphasis on evidence-based practices, insurance companies and schools may not pay for expensive alternative vision treatments that fail to work on broad groups of people. There is a need to research subgroups where these treatments may be beneficial. I have talked to many people, both on and off the spectrum, who have been helped by using tinted glasses and colored paper. Trying on glasses is free and single sheets of 10 different shades of pastel, gray, and tan paper cost only a few cents. I have observed several college students who were saved from flunking out of school with this simple intervention. It will not work for everybody, but it is definitely worth trying.

References

Bakroonm, A. and Lakshminarayanan, V. (2016) Visual function in autism spectrum disorders: A critical review, *Clinical and Experimental Optometry* 99:doi.org/10.1111/exo.12383.

Beasley, I., and N. Davis. 2013. "The Effect of Spectral Filters on Reading Speed and Accuracy Following Stroke." *Journal of Optometry* 6(3):134–40.

Henderson, L., N. Tsogka, and M. Snowling. 2012. "Questioning the Benefits that Coloured Overlays Can Have for Reading in Students with and without Dyslexia." *Journal of Research in Special Education Needs* 13(1):57–65. doi:10.111l/j.1471.3802.2012.01237

Huang, J., X. Zong, A. Wilkins, B. Jenkins, A. Bozoki, and Y. Cao. 2011. "MRI Evidence that Precision Ophthalmic Tints Reduce Cortical Hyperactivation in Migraine." *Cephalalgia* 31(8):925–36. doi: 10.1177/0333102411409076

Kaplan, M., S. Edelson, and J. Seip. 1998. "Behavioral Changes in Autistic Individuals as a Result of Wearing Ambient Transitional Prism Lenses." *Child Psychiatry and Human Development* 29(1):65–76.

Lightstone, A., T. Lightstone, and A. Wilkins. 1999. "Both Coloured Overlays and Coloured Lenses Can Improve Reading Fluency But Their Optimal Chromaticities Differ." *Ophthalmic and Physiological Optics* 19(4):279–85.

Little, J.A. (2018) Vision in autism spectrum disorder: A critical review, *Clinical and Experimental Optometry.* Doi.org/10.1111/exo.12651.

Ludlow, A., E. Taylor-Whiffen, and A. Wilkins. 2012. "Coloured Filters Enhance the Visual Perception of Social Cues in Children with Autism Spectrum Disorders." *ISRN Neurology* (March 4). doi: 10.5402/2012/298098

Ritchie, S., S. Sala, and R. McIntosh. 2011. "Irlen Colored Overlays Do Not Alleviate Reading Difficulties." *Pediatrics* 128:932–38.

Wilkins, A. 2002. "Coloured Overlays and Their Effects on Reading Speed: A Review." *Ophthalmic and Physiological Optics* 22(5):448–54.

When I was little, I could understand what people were saying when they spoke directly to me. But when adults talked fast, it sounded like gibberish.

Auditory Processing Problems and Sound Over Sensitivity in Autism

Anyone who has attended one of my presentations know that it is my opinion that sensory issues are a big part of behavior problems in children with autism. I, myself, have many sensory issues and one that affects me the most is excessive reactions to sudden loud noises.

The U.S. DSM-5 diagnostic guidelines include sensory problems as part of the diagnosis of autism. Unfortunately, the new ICD-11 guideline does not include sensory problems for autism. Fortunately, all diagnostic guidelines include central auditory processing disorder. For insurance purposes, a child's or adult's problems with sound oversensitivity can be diagnosed as auditory processing disorder. Auditory processing problems are often associated with neurodevelopmental disorders such as dyslexia, ADHD, and autism. These problems can be present even though the child is not deaf.

When I was a child, the ringing of the school bell hurt my ears. It felt like a dentist's drill hitting a nerve. This is common among the autism population. The sounds that are most likely to hurt the ears are high-pitched, shrill, intermittent sounds such as fire alarms, smoke detectors, certain ringtones on mobile phones, or the screech of feedback from a microphone. Once a child experiences the pain associated with certain sounds, he/she is not soon to forget it.

Subsequently, a child may have a tantrum and refuse to enter a certain room because he/she may be afraid that the fire alarm might go off, or that the assembly microphone might screech again. Even if it happened months and months ago, and even if it only happened one time, he/she may take action to avoid feeling that pain again. Sometimes sound sensitivity can be desensitized by recording the offending sound and allowing the child to initiate the sounds at gradually increasing volume. It is important for the child to be able to control the sound. A child that fears the sound of the vacuum cleaner may learn to like it if he/she can turn it on and off and control it. Problems with sound sensitivity are very variable. A sound that hurts the ears of one child may be attractive to another. Parents and professionals need to be good detectives and watch for clues from the child about what auditory sounds are troublesome.

A study done with German Shepherd dogs may provide insights into over-sensitivity to sound in autism. Dogs are highly variable in their reactions to sounds. Some dogs are highly fearful of both sudden, loud sounds and novel situations. The genetic factors of these traits are similar in both people and dogs. The dogs with their genetic trait may feel pain in response to sudden loud sounds. In my own case, a sudden loud sound, such as a fire alarm, caused an exaggerated startle reaction. Medication now controls my overall response, but I will have the initial startle.

Auditory Detail Abilities May be Impaired

Even though children and adults with ASD can easily pass a standard hearing test, they often have difficulty hearing auditory detail. When I was little, I could understand what people were saying when the spoke directly to me, but when adults talked fast it sounded like gibberish. All I could hear were the vowels, and I thought that grownups had their own "grownup" language. Children who remain nonverbal may be hearing only the vowels and no consonants.

My speech teacher helped me hear the consonants by stretching them out. She would hold up a cup and ask me to say "c-c-c-u-p-p." She alternated between saying "cup" the normal way and stretching it out. If there was a lot of background noise, I had difficulty hearing. Eye contact is still difficult for me in noisy rooms because it interferes with hearing. My brain's wiring allows only one sense to function at a time. This is especially a problem in noisy environments. In noisy rooms, I have to concentrate on hearing.

As an adult, I took a number of central auditory processing tests and was shocked at how poorly I did. Words like "lifeboat" and lightbulb" were mixed up. I did poorly on the dichotic listening test where I had a man talking in one ear and woman talking in the other ear. When I had to attend to my left ear, I was functionally deaf. However, both of my ears tested normal in the simple hearing threshold test. I also had difficulty discriminating between two short sounds that occurred close together. For example, a one second sound followed by a half second gap and then another one second sound is perceived as a single sound. Normal people can discriminate which sound has a higher pitch, and therefore their brain registers two sounds. I cannot do this because the sounds blend together.

Recent research indicates that people with autism have more nervous system arousal and greater difficulty doing a complex task in a noisy environment.

Parents and teachers working with children with ASD need to be aware of these auditory processing difficulties. Sometimes a child's behavior can be a direct result of his/her lack of auditory processing skills rather than disobedience or what may look like "acting out" behaviors. Imagine how you would (or would not) function if you heard only parts of words, only vowels, or only certain tones. How much important relevant information would you miss every day, every hour, every minute?

There are some kids who can learn to speak by singing. Try singing words to the child. Singing uses different circuits in the brain.

A child who has difficulty hearing auditory detail will benefit from the use of visual supports, such as written words on flashcards, written instructions, or written homework assignments. He/she may need to hear and read the word at the same time for comprehension to take place.

Give the Child Time to Respond

A common mistake is not giving the child sufficient time to respond to a question. The brain of a child with autism is like a slow computer. If he/she is forced to answer quickly, he/she may freeze. The child may take longer to respond than a so-called "normal" child. Be patient and allow extra time for a response.

Another problem in some children is "clipping." When spoken to, the child's auditory system may miss the first few words of the sentence. To prevent this from occurring, get the child's attention first by saying his/her name or some other short phrase. The channel is now open and he/she will be more likely to hear the whole sentence.

References and Additional Reading

Dawes, P. and Bishop, D.V.M. (2010) Psychometric profile of children with auditory processing disorder and children with dyslexia, *Archives Disabled Child*, 95:432-436.

DeWit, E. et al. (2018) Same or different: The overlap between children with auditory processing disorders and children with other developmental disorders: A systematic review, *Ear and Hearing*, 39:1-19.

Heaton, P, Davis, R.E. and Happe, F.G. (2008) Research note: Exceptional absolute pitch perception for spoken words in an able adult with autism, *Neuropsychological* 46:2095-2098.

ICD-10-CM Diagnosis Code H93.25 Central Auditory Processing Disorder Illiandou, V. (2017) A European perspective on auditory processing disorder – Current Knowledge and Future Research Focus, *Frontiers in Neurology*, 8:622.

Johansson, O., and Lindegren, D. (2008) Analysis of everyday sounds which are extremely annoying for children with autism, *Journal of Acoustical Society of America*, 123:3299.

Joosten, A.V. and Bundy, A.C. (2010) Sensory processing and stereotypical and repetitive behavior in children with autism and intellectual disability, *Australia Journal of Occupational Therapy*, 57:366-372.

Keith, J.M. et al. (2019) The influence of noise on autonomic arousal and cognitive performance in adolescents with autism spectrum disorder, *Journal of Autism and Developmental Disorders*, 49:113-126.

Robertson, E.E. and Baron-Cohen, S. (2017) Sensory perception in autism, *Nature Reviews Neuroscience* 18:671-684.

Russo, N.Z. et al. (2009) Effects of background noise on cortical encoding of speech in autism spectrum disorders, *Journal of Autism and Developmental Disorders* 39:1185-1196.

Sarviaho, O. et al. (2019) Two novel genomic regions associated with fearfulness in dogs overlap human neuropsyciatric loci, *Translational Psychiatry* 9(18) www.nature.com/articles/s4/1398-018-0361-x.

Wan, C.Y. et al. (2010) The therapeutic effects of singing in neurological disorders, *Music Perception* 27:287-295.

Incorporating Sensory Methods into Your Autism Program

C hildren and adults with autism spectrum disorders, be they mildly or severely challenged, have one or more of their senses affected to the extent that it interferes with their ability to learn and process information from the world around them. Often, the sense of hearing is the most affected, but vision, touch, taste, smell, balance (vestibular), and awareness of their body in space (proprioception) can all function abnormally in the person with autism. Therefore, I am a strong proponent of sensory integration (SI) as a must-have therapy for this population.

Most school systems have an occupational therapist (OT) who can assess the child's needs, set up a daily "diet" plan, and provide sensory treatment to a child. It is just common sense that sensory integration activities such as relaxing deep pressure, swinging, visual tools, and other strategies be components of any good autism program. These activities help the child's nervous system calm down so the child can be more receptive to learning. They can also help reduce hyperactivity, tantrums, and repetitive stimming, or rev up a lagging system in a child who is hypo-sensitive. SI ensures that a child is at optimal levels of attention and readiness to benefit from other intervention programs, such as behavioral, educational, speech, or social skills programs.

A randomized trial has shown that sensory interventions are effective. This provides evidence-based validation of their methods. To be effective, sensory activities must be done every day.

I still encounter parents and some professionals who believe that SI doesn't work, precisely because the activities have to be repeated on a daily basis. Would you question whether or not eyeglasses worked because they had to be used every day? Another example is using medication to improve behaviors. Medication has to be taken every day in order for it to be effective. The same holds true for sensory activities.

ABA (Applied Behavior Analysis) techniques are the core of many good autism programs. Research clearly shows that a good ABA program using discrete trial is very effective for teaching language to young children with ASD. The best ABA programs carried out today are more flexible than the original Lovaas method, where most of the activities were done while the child was seated at a table. Newer programs have a greater variety of activities, and teaching often takes place in more natural settings. However, even well-trained ABA professionals are frequently bewildered about how to incorporate SI into their behavior-based program. In my opinion, their problem stems from their viewing SI (or any adjunct therapy program) as separate and apart from the ABA program. Therapies for children with autism are interrelated. We can't work just on behavior, or just on social skills, or just on sensory. The progress achieved in one area will affect functioning in another, and all need to be integrated into a whole to achieve maximum benefits. To use a visual analogy: a good ABA program is like a Christmas tree. It is the framework, the foundation, the base of a child's therapeutic program. Because of the differences manifested by people on the spectrum, other adjunct programs are often needed in addition to ABA, like sensory integration, dietary intervention, social skills training, or language therapy. These services are the ornaments on the tree, which render each tree unique, beautiful, and specific to one child's needs and level of functioning.

There are several easy ways to combine sensory integration or the environmental enrichment program described in this section with a young child's behavior-based program. Try doing some discrete trials while the child receives soothing pressure paired with different pleasant odors the child likes. It may be more effective if the odors that are used are changed frequently. Also try pairing different odors with having the child feel a constantly changing variety of textures, ranging from a soft stuffed animal to a coarse towel or carpet. Recent research shows that two sensory systems should be stimulated with stimuli that are changed frequently. One child I knew learned best when he lay across a beanbag chair, and another bag was placed on top of him, sandwich style. The pressure calmed his nervous system and made him ready for learning. Try slow swinging—ten to twelve times a minute—during the lesson. Swinging helps stimulate language and is why a growing number of speech and occupational therapists hold joint therapy sessions to improve learning. To help a fidgety child sit still and attend to his lesson, try a weighted vest. The vest is most effective if the child wears it for twenty minutes and then takes it off for twenty minutes. This prevents habituation. Conversely, rev up a slower sensory system so that learning can happen by doing a drill while a child jumps on a trampoline, or by using a vibrating chair pad. Some of the children with the most severe autism function like a TV with bad reception: visual and auditory perception fade in and out depending on the strength of the signal. In the most severe cases, visual and auditory information is scrambled, rendering the child unable to decipher what he sees or hears at any given moment.

Brain scan studies show that the brain circuits that perceive complex sounds are abnormal. Sensory integration activities may help unscramble the child's perception and enable information to get through—a prerequisite for any type of learning.

While sensory challenges often lessen over time, and especially as a result of SI treatment, we must acknowledge the detrimental effects that sensory impairments have on the ability of children with ASD to benefit from any treatment, and plan accordingly. Sensory integration should be an important part of any treatment program for a person with ASD.

References

Boddart, N. et al. 2004. Perception of complex sounds in autism: Abnormal auditory cortical processing in children. *American Journal of Psychiatry* 161: 2117-2120.

Ray, T.C., L.J. King, and T. Grandin. 1988. The effectiveness of self-initiated vestibular stimulation on producing speech sounds. *Journal of Occupational Therapy Research* 8: 186-190.

Schaaf, R.L., Benevides, T., Mailloux, Z., et al. 2013. In intervention for sensory difficulties in children with autism: a randomized trial. *Journal of Autism and Developmental Disorders* (In press).

Smith, S.A., B. Press, K.P. Koenig, and M. Kinnealey. 2005. Effects of sensory integration intervention on self-stimulating and self-injurious behaviors. *America Journal of Occupational Therapy* 59: 418-425.

Woo, C.C., and Leon, M. 2013. Environmental enrichment as an effective treatment for autism: a randomized controlled trial. *Behavioral Neuroscience*.

Zisserman, L. 1992. The effect of deep pressure on self-stimulating behaviors in a child with autism and other disabilities. *American Journal of Occupational Therapy* 46: 547-551.

The Effect of Sensory and Perceptual Difficulties on Learning Patterns

I ndividuals on the autism spectrum have remarkably varied problems with sensory over-sensitivity and information processing.
While these problems originate in the brain—their source is biological—they manifest in behaviors that compromise the individuals' ability
to learn and function in the world around them. In my analysis of reports
from many people with autism, it appears that the faulty manner in which
their brains process incoming information can be grouped into three basic
categories: 1) sensory oversensitivity; 2) perceptual problems; and 3) difficulties organizing information.

Sensory Oversensitivity

From child to child, sensory oversensitivity is very variable. It can range
from mild (slight anxiety when the environment is too loud, too bright, or
too chaotic) to severe, with an individual going into a screaming tantrum
every time he is in a large supermarket. One child may not tolerate fluorescent lights; another, like me, fears sudden loud noise because it hurts
his ears. Children may be gagged by certain smells such as perfumes. The
taste and/or texture of foods can be repulsive. Light touch can be merely
annoying or actually painful. One child may enjoy water play and splash-
ing and another may run screaming from it. Some individuals on the

spectrum are attracted to objects that move rapidly and others will avoid them. When senses are disordered, the attention and concentration that learning requires become difficult and in some cases, impossible. Children who spend their days fearful of people and places that, through past experience, have been overwhelming to their senses, have little chance to relax enough to take notice of the learning opportunities being presented.

Research involving functional magnetic resonance imaging brain examinations shows that exposure to mildly aversive sounds and visual stimuli will cause greater activation of the primary sensor cortex and the amygdala (fear center) in individuals with autism. The degree of activation is correlated with ratings of sensory problems by parents.

Perceptual Problems

Problems in this category often determine the style of learning that will be most effective. A child with poor auditory perception may hear sound like a bad mobile phone connection, where the voice fades in and out or entire parts of the communication are missing. The child is more likely to learn best with visually presented information. A child with visual perception problems may learn best through the auditory channel. Children who look out the corner of their eye while reading often have visual processing problems. Suspect a visual processing problem in children who finger-flick in front of their eyes, or hate either fluorescent lights or escalators. To some of these individuals, the world looks like it is viewed through a kaleidoscope: flat, without depth perception, and broken into pieces. For others, it is

like looking through a small tube, seeing only the small circle of vision directly in front of them, with no peripheral vision. Some nonverbal individuals have both visual and auditory processing problems. They may learn best through their sense of touch and smell. For instance, to learn to get ready in the morning, they may need to be "walked" through (hand-over-hand) tasks such as putting on socks or pouring cereal. They may learn letters and numbers best when they can touch them, and trace their shape with their hands or fingers. Representative objects rather than visual charts can be useful in helping these individuals know when it is time to transition to a new activity.

Organizing Information

Because of these faulty connections in the brain, an individual may receive information but be unable to organize it or make sense of it. Donna Williams, a well-known person with autism from Australia, mentions that spoken words turn into "blah-blah-blah" and the meaning disappears. She is hearing the words clearly but not understanding them. Problems with organizing information affect children's ability to form categories—the foundation for later concept formation. Difficulties people on the spectrum have with multi-tasking would also fall into this category. Again, these difficulties are highly variable, and range from mild to severe depending on which brain

circuits connected and which ones did not during development. One classic test of flexible thinking is the Wisconsin Card Sorting Test. In this test, a person has to sort differently-patterned cards, one at a time, into categories such as *yellow* or *circles*. A person on the spectrum is slower to figure out new categories as they are introduced.

Sensory overload can cause either vision or hearing to shut down completely. During these times, no information will get through to the brain, and learning will not occur. Also, sensory and information processing problems are worse when a child is tired. It is therefore best to teach difficult material when the child is alert and wide awake. Since my oversensitivity to noise was fairly mild, I responded well to a gently intrusive teaching method where the teacher grabbed my chin to make me pay attention. Donna Williams told me that method absolutely would not work with her. The tactile input coupled with the teacher speaking would be overload and could not be processed simultaneously. Donna is a mono-channel learner. She either has to look at something or listen to something, but she cannot look and listen at the same time. Information processing on more than one sensory channel is not possible.

An effective teacher with spectrum children and adults is one who is a good detective and looks for the source of learning difficulties.

Often they can be found in one or a combination of these categories mentioned above. A challenge, even one considered mild, will dramatically compromise a child's ability to learn via traditional teaching methods. Teachers who truly want to help students with sensory and perception difficulties will figure out the child's unique learning style and adapt teaching methods accordingly. Some children do best with written instructions and assignments; others will do best through oral methods or oral testing. The best teachers have a flexible approach and teach to the style through which each child learns.

References

Gastgeb, H.Z., M.S. Strauss, and N.J. Minshew. 2006. Do individuals with autism process categories differently? The effect of typicality and development. *Child Development* 77: 1717-1729.

Grandin,T. and Panek, R. 2013. *The Autistic Brain*. Houghton Mifflin Harcourt, New York, NY.

Green, SA, et al. 2013. Overactive brain responses to sensory stimuli in youth with autism spectrum disorder. *Journal American Academy of Child and Adolescent Psychiatry* 52:1158-1172.

Lidstone J. 2014. Relations among restricted and repetitive behaviors, anxiety and sensory features in children with autism spectrum disorders, *Research in Autism Spectrum Disorders* 8:82-92

Shulamite A.G. 2015. Neurobiology of Sensory Overresponsivity in Youth With Autism Spectrum Disorders, *JAMA Psychiatry,* doi:10.1001/jama-psychiatry.2015.0737

Environmental Enrichment Therapy for Autism

A simple and easy-to-implement series of environmental enrichment experiences has been shown to greatly reduce the severity
of symptoms in children with autism. The treatment consists of a
variety of sensory exercises that are done for 30 minutes each day. This research was conducted by Cynthia Woo and Michael Leon at the University
of California at Irvine.[1]

The program was designed to use economical and readily available
household materials. Research with animals has clearly shown that combinations of olfactory (smell) and tactile stimulation are very beneficial to
the developing brain. Stimulation of the senses of BOTH smell and touch
with constantly changing stimulation is a foundation of the treatment.
The principle behind the therapy is to always simultaneously stimulate two
or more senses. Another basic principle is NOVELTY ... the stimulation
must be constantly changing. Stimulation of a single sense alone is not
effective.

Patients were assigned to undergo either environmental enrichment
or standard treatment (the control group). All children underwent applied
behavioral analysis (ABA) and speech therapy.

Every day, children received a combination of olfactory stimulation paired with touch stimulation, such as rubbing the back. A different,
pleasant odor was used each day. The odors were essential oils of lemon,
apple, lavender, vanilla, and other appealing scents. Each day, a different

pleasant scent was used. If the child hates one particular scent, then stop using it. Let the child pick a VARIETY of pleasant odors.

In addition to exposure to scents and touch, the treatment consisted of 33 different exercises that gradually increased in difficulty. Each exercise was done for two weeks before going to the next exercise. All exercises stimulated two or more senses at the same time. The exercises are designed to be always varied and increasingly challenging. It is important to NEVER keep doing the same thing.

When the child progressed to the next exercise, there was a change in the pair of senses stimulated. Some examples of the exercises were drawing lines on the child's hands with objects that had different textures (touch and visual stimulation), and warm and cool spoons were used to draw lines on the child's arms while the parent played music (thermal, touch, and auditory stimulation).

Other exercises required walking along a narrow board or identifying objects in a pillowcase by touching them and matching them with the same objects viewed on a table. The exercises become progressively more difficult. The 25th exercise required the child to put coins into a piggy bank by viewing its reflection in a mirror (motor, visual, and cognitive stimulation). The entire research article, with the method clearly explained, can be downloaded for free on the Internet.

At the end of six months, the exercises resulted in great improvements—even in the older children. The authors concluded that 42% of the enriched group improved, but only 7% of the control group improved. A more recent trial showed that when environmental enrichment is done with three to six-yearold children, 21% of the children had dramatic improvement.

Parents and teachers can easily follow the methods described in their two papers. I had the opportunity to visit with Dr. Leon.

He has replicated his research and has found that environmental enrichment is helpful for both young and older children. This therapy is designed to be done in conjunction with standard care, such as ABA and speech therapy. For the complete directions, download the free article. Type the title into Google.

References

www.mendability.com. Accessed June 25, 2019.

Aronoff, E. et al. (2016) Environmental enrichment therapy for autism: Outcomes with increased access, *Neuroplasticity* 2734915, doi:10.1155/2018/2016/2734915.

Padmanabha, H. et al. (2019) Homebased sensory intervention in children with autism spectrum disorder: A randomized controlled trial, *The Indian Journal of Pediatrics*, 86:18-25.

Woo C.C. et al. 2015. Environmental enrichment as a therapy for autism: A clinical trial replication and extension, *Behavior Neuroscience* Vol. 129, pp 412-422.

Woo, C.C. and Leon, M. 2013 Environmental enrichment as an effective treatment for autism: A randomized controlled trial. *Behavior Neuroscience*. DOI: 10.1037/a0033010.

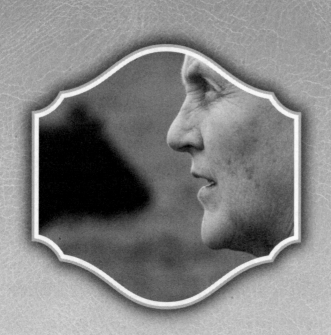

CHAPTER 4

Understanding Nonverbal Autism

*These individuals are highly aware
of their surroundings and have self
learned far more than parents and
teachers imagine. It's their bodies that
don't work, not their minds.*

To understand the mind of a child or adult who is completely nonverbal, without oral, signed, written, or typed language, you must leave the world of thinking in words. This can be quite challenging for many people. Our society functions through the spoken word. For the majority of people, words are their "native language." It is difficult for them to step outside this very basic way of relating and imagine something else. Some neurotypical people, especially those with stronger creative sides, can do this. Other neurotypical people struggle immensely in understanding this concept.

I think in pictures. It's been that way forever for me. When I was very young, before any speech or language training, there were no words in my head. Now, words narrate the pictures in my imagination, but pictures remain my primary "language."

For a minute, try to imagine an inner world of picture-based or sensory-based thoughts. The closest analogy that may make sense to most neurotypical people who think in words is to recall a recent dream. Many dreams do not contain language. They are flowing sequences of pictures, with associated emotional impressions. Sometimes these pictorial narrations make sense, and we come away with a "message" from the dream.

Many times, the images are strange and disconnected from one another, and we awake, scratching our heads and wondering, "What was that dream all about?" If the nonverbal person has a severe visual processing problem, now imagine that your visual system is providing jumbled images, like a pixelated video screen with a poor satellite signal. All the common sounds that most people ignore, such as the sound of people walking or doors opening and closing, cannot be filtered out. This is what a nonverbal person may face. Hearing individual conversations may be difficult and may be like struggling with a mobile phone with a weak signal.

To imagine a nonverbal person's world, I shut my eyes and think with each of my individual senses. What would thinking in touch be like, if I cannot rely on the distorted input from my dysfunctional visual and auditory systems? How might I function if I could only relate to my world through my sense of smell? As an exercise in touch and smell thought, the reader could think about a vacation on the beach. There are usually vivid impressions of the color and sound of the ocean, the feel of the warm sand, and the salty smell. When a nonverbal person thinks or daydreams, maybe there are no words going through his head.

There are only sensory impressions, such as images, sounds, smells, touch, and taste sensations coming into his consciousness. If the person has severe problems with both visual and auditory processing, his brain may rely on his other senses to make sense of his world. His only coherent thoughts may be in touch, taste, or smell sensations. These forms of sensory input may be the only way he obtains accurate information about his environment. Maybe this is why some nonverbal individuals touch, tap, and smell things. It's how they learn about their world. Our typical way of life, and especially our education system, is largely based on visual and auditory sharing of information.

Imagine how difficult mere existence would be if those information channels were constantly turned off or if they functioned poorly in an individual. Parents, teachers, and therapists need to be good detectives in working with nonverbal individuals to figure out which senses are working best. For some, the auditory sense is preferred, and for others, it's vision. For a minority of people, the sense of touch may be the primary learning channel. A basic principle is to use the sensory system that works the best. However, this will be highly variable among different nonverbal individuals.

Nonverbal, with or without Cognitive Impairment

The reader may wonder where I concocted all these ideas about nonverbal people's perceptions. They are based on neuroscience knowledge, coupled with reports from many verbal individuals who can describe their very severe sensory problems. Many individuals who have more severe sensory problems than mine describe sensory scrambling or the shutdown of one or more senses. This occurs more frequently when the individuals are tired or in a highly stimulating environment, such as a large supermarket. Included in this section are three articles about Tito and Carly. They are nonverbal individuals who can type independently and, in striking detail, describe their inner world. Tito has written about disordered, jumbled visual perceptions.

He also described a thinking self that exists separate from an acting self. He cannot control some of his flapping movements. His mind and body are not integrated together. The human   brain contains circuits for color, shape, and motion. These circuits have to work together to form images. Tito describes visual perception where it is obvious that these circuits are not working together. He may see the color of an object before he can identify it by shape. For parents and teachers who work with nonverbal individuals, I strongly recommend Tito's book, *How Can I Talk If My Lips Don't Move?* Two other books that will provide great insight into the world of nonverbal people with autism are *The Reason I Jump*, by Noaki Higashida, and *Carly's Voice*. All three of these individuals can use a keyboard without anyone having to touch them. If somebody is holding the child's arm or wrist, this person may be the author of the child's writing.

As a society, we equate intelligence with language. Smart people are verbal people. The verbal people who can express themselves best are assumed to be most intelligent. People who can't use language well are perceived as dumb. We don't usually stop and question whether oral-motor skills, rather than intelligence, might be causing the language impairment. No, we do just the opposite and almost instantaneously judge the nonverbal person as being mentally impaired. Poor guy—he can't talk. And, in our minds, we continue with the most damaging thought of all: *He must not have anything to say.*

This is very true within the autism community. We assume that those who are nonverbal, especially children who have been nonverbal since birth, have reduced or limited cognitive abilities. Many professionals believe that 75% of these individuals function at a mentally retarded level, based on IQ scores. This sets up a vicious cycle: We expect less from these kids, so they receive fewer opportunities to learn. We don't challenge them to learn because we've already decided that they can't. We test these children for IQ, using testing instruments that are largely ill suited to this population, and then point to their low scores as confirmation of impaired mental functioning.

The way I see it, it's time we rethink nonverbal individuals with autism and realize that the preconceived notions we've been using to relate to and educate this population over the   past 20 years are flat-out wrong. Luckily, other professionals in the autism community are coming to the same conclusion, and research is shedding light on the hidden abilities within this population. Professionals have generally agreed that about 50% of individuals with autism will never speak. Catherine Lord, a University of Michigan pioneer in autism research, is suggesting we may be way off the mark. In her 2004 study sample of children who received a diagnosis and began undergoing treatment at age two, only 14% remained nonverbal by age nine, and 35%45% could speak fluently.

Our current perceptions about nonverbal individuals with autism are also being stretched by people on the spectrum, like Tito, Carly Fleischman, Naoki Higashida, and others, who are coming forth and writing about their rich inner worlds and their abilities. Bit by bit, they are deflating the notion that not being able to speak means not having anything to say. Through the increased use of augmentative and alternative communication aids with nonverbal individuals, we are discovering that many children with autism have taught themselves to read. These individuals are highly aware of their surroundings and have selflearned far more than parents and teachers imagine. It's their bodies that don't work, not their minds.

Carly Fleischman describes having great difficulty with filtering out environmental sensory input. She is a normal teenage girl locked in a body she has difficulty controlling. Naoki Higashida describes being embarrassed by uncontrollable movements. Both Tito and Carly have to exert great effort to block out extraneous stimuli and pay attention. When I visited Tito, he could answer only three questions before he needed to rest. iPads and other tablet computers have helped many nonverbal individuals. Typing is easier for them on a table, because the typed letter on the virtual keyboard appears right next to the keyboard. The individual does not need to shift his gaze to see the letter. Shifting his gaze between the keyboard and a desktop or laptop screen is very difficult.

And, these individuals have a lot to say. Amanda Baggs is one such woman, and her 9-minute YouTube clip, "In My Language," is illuminating to all who watch it. As it opens, we see her rocking back and forth, flapping her hands in front of a large window. She goes through a series of odd repetitive behaviors, all the while accompanied by an almost eerie hum. She swats at a necklace with her hand, slaps a sheet of paper against a window, runs her hand over a computer keyboard, and flicks a metal band against a doorknob. Then the words "A Translation" appear on the screen, and the 27-year-old nonverbal autistic woman mesmerizes us with a highly articulate explanation of her thoughts and her actions. She explains how touch, taste, and small provide her with a "constant conversation" with her environment. She challenges our neurotypical way of thinking about nonverbal individuals in a manner that cannot be ignored. And I, for one, applaud her and others who are speaking out about what it means, and doesn't mean, to be nonverbal and have autism. It's about time.

In our interactions with nonverbal individuals with autism, it is critical that we accurately determine their level of ability and challenge and not automatically make assumptions based on their verbal language capabilities or their IQ scores. It is true that many highly impaired individuals with autism exist who also have accompanying mental retardation. But, that percentage may be far less than what we currently assume. When a person who is nonverbal acquires the ability to use language, it changes his life. Tito told me that before he could type, he had "emptiness." It appears that in some cases, nonverbal autism is a "locked-in syndrome," where a normal mind is trapped in a sensory and motor system that does not work. I hypothesize that nonverbal autism is very different than fully verbal ASD. Fully verbal ASD may be more of a lack of social-emotional relatedness, and nonverbal individuals may have more normal emotional systems locked in by faulty sensory systems. There is further information on sensory oversensitivity in chapter 3 and in my book *The Autistic Brain*.

Slow Processing of Information

For most nonverbal and impaired individuals with ASD, the brain processes information very slowly. They may have fewer input channels open to receive information, or their connections may work like a dial-up rather than a high-speed Internet connection. They need much more time to switch gears between different tasks. In autism and many other developmental disorders, attention shifting is slow, and nonverbal impaired individuals are often slower than individuals with milder forms of autism. In her lectures, Lorna King, one of the early pioneers in using sensory integration, warned all therapists attending her meetings about a phenomenon called "clipping." Clipping can occur in individuals who are both verbal and nonverbal. Attention shifting can be so slow that the person may miss half the information the teacher is trying to convey to them. This is most likely to happen when the child's attention has to be shifted to a new task. For example, if I said to a child playing with his toy, "The juice is on the table," the child may hear only "on the table." To avoid this problem, the parent or teacher should first capture the child's attention with a phrase like, "Tommy, I need to tell you something." Then deliver the instruction or important information. If half of that first phrase is "clipped," it does not matter, because now the input channel is open, and the statement about the juice can get through.

Fear Is the Main Emotion

All behavior occurs for a reason. When a nonverbal impaired person has a tantrum, fear may be the main motivator. There   is now functional magnetic resonance imaging evidence that sensory oversensitivity is associated with increased activation of the amygdala (the fear center in the brain). In my own case, small high-pitched noises that occur at night still set off a little twinge of fear in me. The big, heart-pounding, fearful reactions I used to have during my 20s are now controlled with antidepressant drugs. Trying to eliminate these big-fear reactions through cognitive or behavioral methods didn't work for me. Self-reports from other individuals also indicate that certain sounds or sensations cause panic attacks. Recently, brain imaging at the University of Utah showed that the amygdala in my brain is enlarged. This may explain my increased fear responses. If an individual is nonverbal and his receptive learning is impaired, harmless things such as a certain room or a particular person may be associated with a stimulus that hurts, such as a smoke alarm. In some cases, the individual might associate the dreadful sound with something he was looking at when the alarm went off. If he was looking at a teacher's blue jacket, he may develop a blue-jacket fear. I know this sounds odd, but these associative fear memories occur all the time in animals. A dog often fears the place where he got hit by a car instead of being afraid of cars. If these associations can be figured out, it may be possible to remove the feared object. I discuss fear memories in more depth in my book, *Animals in Translation*.

An individual with severe autism can easily panic if something new is suddenly introduced. A surprise birthday party can trigger a tantrum instead of pleasure. It is best to gradually habituate the child to the things he or she will experience at the party. This is very similar to habituating horses to tolerate the new, scary things they will see at a horse show. They need to gradually get used to new things such as flags and balloons at home, before they go to a show. Individuals with severe autism can learn to like new things. The best way to introduce them is to let the child or adult gradually approach and explore them at his or her own pace and inclination. Some nonverbal individuals may explore them by touching, smelling, or tasting. They need to be provided with a specific place where they are allowed to do this kind of exploration, because licking things at the grocery store is not appropriate behavior. Nonverbal impaired people are usually able to learn that certain activities are only allowed in certain places. For instance, if the person does not want to taste a new food, he or she may need to explore it first by touching or smelling it. This activity should be done away from the dining room because touching and smearing food is not appropriate behavior in the dining room.

Self-Injurious Behavior (SIB)

Some nonverbal individuals, and even some highly verbal individuals, engage in banging their heads or biting themselves. Reports form people on the spectrum have revealed that many of these problems stem from severe sensory issues. In this case, the child may be hyposensitive—lacking in sensory input—rather than the more typical hypersensitivity (too much input) that is often the case within the autism population. In some of these cases, individuals do not realize they are being self-injurious because they have tactile or body boundary issues. For example, when they are tired or upset, they cannot determine where their foot ends and the floor begins. They may not feel themselves sitting on a chair at school, so they squirm or bounce in the chair to induce the sensory input they need to feel stable.

Lorna King found that a child who self-abuses often feels no pain. Children may dig at their skin to the point of drawing blood because their sensory receptors return no tactile sensation, as would happen in a typical person. After King introduced children to activities that provided calming sensory stimulation, such as deep pressure or slow swinging, pain sensation returned. She has seen children who used to bang their heads start to hit their heads and stop before they did so, because they know it will hurt now. You may also want to try the environmental enrichment method of pairing different odors with different textures for the child to touch. See the chapter on environmental enrichment for more information. (See the chapter "Solving Behavior Problems in Nonverbal Individuals with Autism" for information on hidden painful medical problems that may cause self-abuse.) For some severe cases of SIB, treatment with the opiate-blocking drug Naltrexone may be helpful. There is an excellent open-access article by Dr. Sandman and Dr. Kemp from the University of California in the reference list.

The best approach for controlling SIB is an integrated approach. A combination of behavioral analysis, sensory therapy, conventional medications, and biomedical interventions, such as diets and supplements, often works best. The big mistake that many people make when treating SIB is to get too single-minded in their approach. Some people try to use just behavioral analysis and never use a drug. Others use drugs and nothing else. Both single-minded approaches are wrong. A drug-only approach leads to a case of a sleepy "drug zombie," and a behavioral-only approach without any intervention to reduce nervous system arousal may lead to the use of bad procedures, such as long periods of restraint.

Does the Nonverbal Person Understand Speech?

In some cases, nonverbal people have receptive language and can understand what is being said. In other cases, they do not. Nonverbal people are masters at reading slight differences in a teacher's or parent's actions. I had one parent tell me that her child has ESP, because he is already waiting at the door before his mother even gets her car keys or purse. It is likely that the individual is sensing slight differences in behavior before it's time to get the keys or purse. There may be some hustle and bustle activities, such as throwing out the newspaper. If the child has severe visual processing problems, he may be responding to the sounds of the paper being crushed in the trashcan.

In some situations, the nonverbal individual may be responding to a gesture rather than a word. If you point to the juice or turn your head toward it, the person may perceive your actions. One way to test receptive language is to ask the person to do something odd. An example would be to ask the child to put his or her book on the chair. In some nonverbal individuals, verbal language is impossible, but they learn to read and express themselves through typing. Their speech circuits are scrambled, but they can still communicate through the typed word.

References

Fleischman, A., Fleischman, C. 2012. *Carly's Voice: Breaking Through Autism*. New York, NY: Touchstone Books.

Fouse, B., Wheeler, M. 1997. *A Treasure Chest of Behavioral Strategies for Individuals with Autism*. Arlington, TX: Future Horizons.

Grandin, T., Johnson, C. 2005. *Animals in Translation*. New York, NY: Scribner.

Grandin, T., Panek, R. 2013. *The Autistic Brain*. New York, NY: Houghton Mifflin Harcourt.

Higashida, N. and Mitchell, D. (2017) *Fall down 7 times, Get up 8, A Young Man's Voice From the Silence of Autism*, Random House, New York.

Horvath, K., Perman, J.A. 2002. Autism and gastrointestinal symptoms. *Current Gastroneurology Reports* 4:251-258.

Kern, J.K., et al. 2007. Sensory correlations in autism. *Autism* 11:123-134.

Muchopadhyay, T.J. (2011) *How Can I Talk if my Lips Don't Move*, Available as Amazon Kindle and audiobook.

Sandman, C.A., Kemp, A.S. 2011. Opioid antagonists may reverse endogenous opiate dependence in treatment of self injurious behavior. *Pharmaceuticals* 4:366-381.

Savarese, R.J. 2007. *Reasonable People: A Memoir of Autism and Adoption—On the Meaning of Family and the Politics of Neurological Difference*. New York, NY: Other Press. (This book describes successful teaching strategies for teaching nonverbal people to type).

Schaller, S. 1995. *A Man without Words*. Berkeley, CA: University of California Press.

Schumann, C.M., et al. 2009. Amygdala enlargement in toddlers with autism related to severity of social and communication impairments. *Biological Psychiatry* 66:942-943.

Williams, D. 1996. *Autism: An Inside-Out Approach*. London, England: Jessica Kingsley Publishers.

Wolfgang, A., Pierce, L., Teder-Salejarvi, W. A., Courchesne, E., Hillyard, S.A. 2005. Auditory spatial localization and attention deficits in autistic adults. *Cognitive Brain Research* 23:221-234.

Wolman, D. 2008. The truth about autism: scientists reconsider what they think they know. *Wired Magazine*, 16:03.

A Social Teenager Trapped Inside

S ome individuals with autism who appear to be low-functioning have a good mind trapped inside a dysfunctional body that they cannot control. Carly Fleischmann appeared to have no skills at all when she was a child. She had no speech, and she was either in constant motion, destroying things, or sitting alone rocking. The only thing she seemed to care about was potato chips. When she was given a device that had pictures that spoke words when pressed, she quickly learned how to use it. But she found it difficult to press the button for a really needed bathroom break when the button for potato chips was so enticing.

Teachers sometimes underestimate a child's abilities. One teacher was going to delete the keyboard function on Carly's communication device. If this had happened, Carly's parents would have never learned that she knew words. One day Carly typed, "Help teeth hurt." After this happened a program was started to teach her more words. Every object in the house was labeled. It turned out that Carly was taking in lots of information even though she appeared to not be paying attention.

As Carly slowly became literate, she explained how typing required great effort. She was extremely anxious, and often she would type only with people she knew. Today Carly is typing independently, and she attends a gifted program at her local public high school. She explains how it was so difficult to control her body and sit still. Unlike me, Carly was interested in boys, movie stars, and all the things that a typical teenage girl would be infatuated with. When she was on national TV, she knew she would have to remain still and have no outbursts. She said it would be easier if the cameraman was really cute. To Carly, autism does not define who she is. She wishes her brain and body could be fixed so that normal activities would be easier.

Sensory Bombardment

Carly thinks in pictures that rush at her all at once. I can control the images that come into my mind, but Carly cannot. Filtering out background stimulation is difficult for Carly, and she often has a hard time understanding what other people are saying.

Carly eloquently describes how sensory stimuli would intrude and make listening to a conversation difficult. Carly reports that she often heard only one or two words in each sentence. She describes how cascades of many different stimuli blocked out the conversation. For example, when she was in a quiet coffee shop talking to another person, the relatively low background noise and visual stimuli of the coffee shop could be filtered out. She calls this "audio filtering," which is often very difficult. Her ability to audio filter became overloaded when a person passed by her table with strong perfume. Now the previously blocked out sounds of the coffee maker and the sight of a door opening and closing all rush in and block out the conversation.

Carly is able to audio filter when the background stimulation is low, but when her audio filtering is overloaded, stimuli from all her senses cascade into her brain and turn everything to chaos. At this point controlling a meltdown is almost impossible.

To help control meltdowns and body movements, Carly does have to take medication. To control herself requires both intense willpower and medication. When she was young, potato chips were the motivation. Today, being able to participate in typical girl interests is the motivator to control her body.

What Is Autism?

Carly's story makes one think, what is autism? In my case autism is part of who I am, and I do not have the social interests that Carly has. I have no desire to change my brain or be cured. At the so-called high end of the spectrum, autism may be a disorder of the social circuits in the brain. At the other end of the spectrum, it may be a "locked in" disorder where a social person is trapped inside a dysfunctional body and sensory system.

I need to warn the reader to be realistic. Not every child on the more severe end of the spectrum can be Carly, but teachers and parents who are observant can see glimpses of true intelligence in individuals who are unable to "speak."

Resource

Fleischmann, A., and C. Fleischmann. 2012. *Carly's Voice*. New York: Touchstone.

A good teacher has good instincts and knows how much a child has to be pushed to get progress.

You Asked Me!

P arents and teachers frequently ask me questions about the child or the student(s) with whom they work. Following are a few of the questions I have been asked repeatedly. I hope they prove informative and useful to your own situation.

—Temple

Q: My nine-year-old son is well-behaved when he is with me (his mom) but screams, kicks, and tears his books at school. What causes this?

A: When I was nine, maintaining a consistent environment at both home and school prevented this problem. I knew that if I misbehaved at school there would be consequences when I got home. A tantrum at school always resulted in loss of watching TV for one night (taking it away for a month would seem like five years to a nine-year-old). When I got home, mother would calmly tell me that Mrs. Dietch had called, so no TV. I knew what the rule was.

There are a lot of possible reasons for behavior problems at school. The foremost cause that needs to be ruled out (or addressed!) is overstimulation from fluorescent lights, and noises, such as the school bell. Loud noises hurt the ears of many children with autism. A child may have a tantrum in the classroom because he never knows when the dreaded fire alarm might go off. If sensory problems are not a part of the behavior problem, it may be that the child is testing you (like most nine-year-olds will); adhering to prescribed rules is more important than ever if this is the case. Last, not every child enjoys school; the child may simply not want to be there. Again, consistent actions and expectations on your part will help immensely. It is important to make sure you tell your son what the rules are and what behaviors you expect of him.

Q: Do rituals and stereotypes differ from obsessive-compulsive behavior?

A: There are several different motivations for the repetitive behavior in children with autism. I needed to dribble sand through my hands to screen out loud sounds that hurt my ears. I would tune out the world. Fortunately, my teachers did not allow me to tune the world out. A second motivation for repetitive behaviors is sudden sensory overload. For instance, a child may suddenly flap his arms when he enters a large supermarket. A third motivation is a neurological tic. This is most likely to occur in nonverbal adults. In some cases the person has little or no voluntary control over the movement.

Obsessive compulsive disorder (OCD) involves repetitive behavior that occurs on a less primitive level. In non-autistic adults, OCD often manifests itself as washing one's hands over and over or constantly checking to see if the doors are locked. Some researchers believe that OCD is caused by a malfunction in the brain circuits that motivate hygiene and checking for danger. These are old, primitive circuits that humans share with animals.

Another repetitive behavior is perseveration. I used to ask the same question over and over. I asked my grandfather a hundred times "Why is the sky blue?" I enjoyed hearing his answer. Perseveration and OCD are probably related. Both behaviors are often alleviated by medications such as Prozac. When I took antidepressants when I was 31, my tendency to perseverate on one topic was greatly reduced. In me, antidepressants reduced anxiety. Reducing anxiety helped to reduce perseveration. From a social perspective, I also had to learn that other people were bored when I discussed the same topics over and over.

Q: *How does a teacher know how much to "push" a child to get progress?*

A: A good teacher has good instincts and knows how much a child has to be pushed to get progress. Part of this skill comes through keen observation and paying close attention to both   the child's interior and exterior world. My speech teacher would grab my chin to make me pay attention. She could kind of yank me out of my autistic world. If she pushed too hard I had a tantrum and if she did not push enough, I made no progress. She had to be "gently insistent." I was a child with relatively mild sensory processing problems. I responded well to a "get in my face" method.

A child with more severe sensory processing problems may go into sensory shut down if a teacher grabs his chin. The child will make more progress if the teacher talks quietly. Children's learning styles vary widely, especially children on the autism spectrum. For one type of child the teacher can "yank open their front door"; for the other type of child, the teacher must "sneak quietly in their back door."

Why Do Kids with Autism Stim?

"S tims" is short for self-stimulatory behaviors, behaviors most people exhibit. We might twirl our hair or tap a pencil—that's stimming. The difference between acceptable stims and those we consider inappropriate is in the type and intense repetition of the stims.

When I did stims such as dribbling sand through my fingers, it calmed me down. When I stimmed, sounds that hurt my ears stopped. Most kids with autism do these repetitive behaviors because it feels good in some way. It may counteract an overwhelming sensory environment, or alleviate the high levels of internal anxiety these kids typically feel every day. Individuals with autism exhibit a variety of stims; they may rock, flap, spin themselves or items such as coins, pace, hit themselves, or repeat words over and over (verbal stims). When these behaviors are uncontrollable, occur excessively in inappropriate settings, or prevent a child from socially acceptable interaction, a problem exists.

A common question both parents and teachers ask me is: "Should the child be allowed to do stims?" My answer is usually "yes and no."

I was allowed to stim in the privacy of my bedroom for one hour after lunch and for a short period of time after dinner. The rest of the time stims were not allowed. Stimming was absolutely forbidden at the dining table, in stores, and in church. I think it is important for a child with autism to have some scheduled time to do stims in private. When they get over stimulated, it helps them calm down. In individuals with more severe autism, stimming can be used as a reward. In some of these individuals, they can sustain attention for very short periods and then need to stim to refocus and realign their systems.

Three Types of Repetitive Behavior

Not all repetitive behaviors are stims, so it is important to distinguish the source behind the behavior.

1. ***Stimming Behaviors.*** These behaviors self-soothe a child and help him regain emotional balance. Unfortunately, if children are allowed to stim all day, no learning will take place because the child's brain is shut off from the outside world. It is perfectly fine to give a child some time to stim but the rest of the day, a young two to five-year-old should be getting three to four hours a day of one-to-one contact with a good teacher to keep the child's brain open to receiving information and learning.

2. ***Involuntary Movements.*** These movements can resemble stims but they may be caused by either Tourette Syndrome or a condition called tardive dyskinesia, which is a side effect of antipsychotic drugs such as Risperal (risperadone), Seroquel (quetiapine) or Abilify (aripiprazole). Nerve damage—sometimes permanent—from these drugs causes the repetitive behaviors. Even though they are approved by the FDA for five-year-olds, they are a poor choice due to the danger of nerve damage and huge weight gain. I would recommend trying a special diet or fish oil supplement first.

3. ***Total Meltdown Due to Sensory Overload.*** When this happens, the child is often having a tantrum while exhibiting repetitive behaviors like kicking or flapping. The best approach is to put the

child in a quiet place and let him calm down. Teaching is impossible during a meltdown. When I was finished having a tantrum, Mother quietly told me the consequence was no TV tonight and that was it.

Depending on the reason for the stimming, therapeutic approaches such as ABA, environmental modifications, or sensory based therapies can be helpful in alleviating or modifying the stim. Parents can also teach the child to substitute a more acceptable behavior for the stim when outside the home, such as rubbing a small object in the child's pocket or squeezing a cushy ball instead of hand flapping.

When I asked him what his life was like before he learned to type, he responded with the word "empty."

Tito Lives in a World of Sensory Scrambling

I n a previous article, I discussed the importance of incorporating sensory integration into the treatment program for a person with ASD. In this anecdote, a real-life example illustrates how far-reaching can be the impact of sensory impairment in a child's life.

I first met Tito Mukhopadhyay* in a quiet medical library. He looked like a typical nonverbal, low-functioning teenager with autism. When he

---

*At the age of three, Tito Mukhopadhyay was diagnosed with severe autism, but his mother, Soma, refused to accept the conventional wisdom of the time that her son would be unable to interact with the outside world. She read to him, taught him to write in English, and challenged him to write his own stories. The result of their efforts is a remarkable book, *The Mind Tree: A Miraculous Child Breaks the Silence of Autism*, written when Tito was between eight and eleven years old. It comprises a broad collection of profound and startling philosophical writings about growing up under the most challenging of circumstances, and how it feels to be locked inside an autistic body and mind. Tito has another book that will provide tremendous insight into how Tito lives in a world of sensory fragmentation.

Another fantastic story is *The Reason I Jump*. People who work with children and adults who remain nonverbal should read all three books that are in the reference list. These three books are all written by nonverbal individuals. They will give you insight into a world of sensory scrambling.

entered the room, he picked up a bright yellow journal and smelled it. He then ran around and flapped.

His mother pulled him over to the computer where I sat and invited me to ask Tito a question about autism. I told her I wanted to ask him about something different, where cueing or prior memorization of an answer would be impossible. From the bottom of a nearby pile of magazines I found an old *Scientific American*. As I thumbed through the magazine I found an illustration of an astronaut riding a horse. When I showed Tito the picture he quickly typed "Apollo II on a horse." This convinced me there was a good brain trapped inside Tito's dysfunctional body.

At a recent conference in Canada, I had another opportunity to talk with Tito. Throughout our conversation, his mother had to keep prompting him to attend to the computer and respond to my questions. I was curious about his sensory systems, so I asked him what his vision was like. He said he saw fragments of color, shapes, and motion. This is a more severe version of the fragmented perception that Donna Williams has described in her books. When I asked him what his life was like before he learned to type, he responded with the word "empty." Despite intervention, Tito still has a very short attention span. He could type only a few short sentences while we were together before he succumbed to sensory overload.

Visual processing challenges such as Tito experiences may stem from abnormal brain connections, according to Dr. Eric Courchesne. The brain has three types of visual perception circuits, each different for color, shape, and motion. In the typical brain, these circuits work together to merge the three visual components into a stable image. Research has shown that in autism there is a lack of interconnections between different parts of the brain. Dr. Eric Courchesne suggests that in autistic brains, large neurons that integrate different brain systems together are abnormal. He states that autism may be an unusual disconnection disorder.

Not all nonverbal children with autism can be like Tito, but he is a prime example of a person with a part of the brain having many broken connections with the outside world. Because of their fragmented abilities, it is important that parents and professionals introduce different modes of communication and social connection, like the keyboard, to children with ASD at an early age so that another Tito is not trapped in emptiness.

References

Courchesne, E. 2004. Brain development in autism: Early overgrowth followed by premature arrest of growth. *Mental Retardation and Developmental Disabilities* 10: 106-111.

Fleishmann, A., and Fleishmann, C. 2012. *Carly's Voice: Breaking Through Autism*. New York, NY: Touchstone Books.

Higashida, N. and Mitchell, D. 2013. *The Reason I Jump: The Inner Voice of a Thirteen Year Old Boy with Autism*. New York, NY: Random House.

Mukhopadhyay, T. 2008. *How Can I Talk If My Lips Don't Move?* New York, NY: Arcade Publishing.

The more we learn about the inner mind of individuals with severe autism, the better able we become to accurately gauge their many abilities and help them achieve their hidden potential.

Understanding the Mind of a Nonverbal Person with Autism

While huge advances have been made over the last few years in understanding "higher functioning" individuals with autism/Asperger's, we still know quite little about the world of the more severely affected individual with autism. In 2007, Tito Mukhopadhyah wrote a book titled *The Mind Tree* that opened the mind of a nonverbal boy with severe autism to the world. Tito's new book *How Can I Talk If My Lips Don't Move?* is equally compelling, highly informative, and should be required reading for everybody who works with nonverbal individuals with autism.

Presumed Intelligence

Tito's mother Soma was a brilliant teacher. She invented all kinds of innovative ways to teach her nonverbal, profoundly autistic son to write and type without assistance. Right from the beginning, Soma assumed Tito was not stupid, so she exposed her young child to many interesting things. She also read to him constantly. She read him children's books and adult books such as Plato, Keats, history, and geometry. When she played with him on a swing she explained the physics of a pendulum. She also took him to many interesting places such as the outdoor food market, other people's houses, and the train station. Even though Tito had all the characteristics of a person with low functioning autism, he was absorbing large amounts of knowledge. Soma instinctively knew that she needed to fill his brain with information.

Sensory Jumble and Panic

Tito's sensory world was a jumble of colors, sounds, and smells. Hearing was his dominant sense and his mother's voice reading to him became a familiar sound that provided order in the chaos. Any little changes in his routine caused panic and a temper tantrum. Tito describes flicking the lights on and off because it brought order to the overwhelming, scattered jumble of sensory overload. Tito is monochannel and he can only attend to one sense at a time. Seeing and hearing at the same time is impossible and his best learning occurs in the morning before he gets tired.

Anything new was totally frightening because the feeling, sight, or sound of a new object was so intense it caused sensory overload and panic. Soma slowly introduced new things and Tito gradually learned to tolerate them. When he got overwhelmed, Tito explained how flapping calmed him down and made him happy. If he had been allowed to do it all day he would have never learned anything. Small amounts of "stimming" were allowed so he could calm down.

Tito Hates Unfinished Tasks and Things

Soma figured out how to motivate completion of a task by doing part of it and then leaving a part unfinished to motivate Tito to finish it. She used a hand-over-hand technique to teach skills such as putting on a shirt, putting on shoes, and how to hold a pencil. Touch provided Tito with more reliable information than vision. To teach a task such as putting on a T-shirt, she placed her hands over his hands and "walked" his hands through the entire task. Gradually she left more and more of the task unfinished so Tito had to finish it. For example, she stopped helping when his arms were through the sleeves and the shirt was half-way over his head. Tito had to pull the shirt the rest of the way himself. This teaching had to be done slowly over several months so Tito's motor memory would learn the entire task.

Difficulty Naming Objects

A psychologist testing Tito could mistakenly think he could not name common objects. He can but he must do it in a roundabout, associative manner. His mind is totally associative. To retrieve the name of an object, he has to be given time to find the word in his memory by providing the definition of the word. Writing the definition enables his associative way of thinking to find the word. When shown a picture of a flower, he is not able to simply say "flower." He has to say, "A soft-petaled part of a plant is a flower." Tito was able to write this definition because he had been exposed to words such as petal. Soma constantly showed him interesting things and pointed to the parts and named them.

This wonderful book will provide parents, educators, and everybody who works with nonverbal individuals insights that will help them work more effectively with this population. Dr. Margaret Bauman, Neurologist at Massachusetts General Hospital emphasizes that we wrongly assume that 75% of nonverbal individuals are mentally retarded. The more we learn about the inner mind of individuals with severe autism, the better able we become to accurately gauge their many abilities and help them achieve their hidden potential.

References

Mukhopadhyah, Tito Rajarshi. 2008. *How Can I Talk If My Lips Don't Move?* New York: Arcade Publishing.

If a functional communication system has not been put into place with a child, his only recourse is behavior.

Solving Behavior Problems in Nonverbal Individuals with Autism

Behavior problems in nonverbal individuals with autism are often difficult to alleviate because these people cannot tell you how they feel. However, all behavior is communication. As a parent, educator, or caregiver, you have to learn to be a good detective to figure out why a nonverbal person with autism is acting out.

If a nonverbal individual who is generally calm suddenly becomes aggressive or frequent tantrums arise, first look for a hidden painful medical problem. Some of the common sources are ear infections, a bad toothache, a sinus infection, gastro-intestinal problems, acid reflux (heartburn), and constipation. You need to be observant; the individual may touch or clutch at the area of the body that hurts, avoid certain foods they previously enjoyed, or their sleep patterns may be different. Acid reflux is common in ASD and stomach pain may explain why a nonverbal individual may refuse to lie down or sit still.

Sensory overload is a second—and more frequent—cause of behavior outbursts. A tantrum in Wal-Mart or other such crowded stores is usually due to sensory overstimulation. Behavior tantrums at school may arise during or prior to times when many students are gathered together, such as recess, lunchtime, or assemblies. Stimuli that are most likely to cause problems are the flicker of fluorescent lights, perfumes/colognes and other strong smells (the cafeteria at school, the store's bakery or seafood section, the restaurant's kitchen), and high-pitched sounds such as squeaky wheels on shopping carts, store product announcements, or smoke alarms. An individual who had previously been calm or cooperative may be afraid to go into a store or a room where a microphone once had audio feedback and squealed. A place that he previously liked may now be too scary because of the association with noxious stimuli. Sounds, smells, and textures that are merely annoying to typical people may be like a dentist's drill hitting a nerve for a person with autism. I have difficulty tolerating scratchy clothes, but for some more sensitive individuals, scratchy sweaters, stiff new clothes, or double-stitched seams may cause a pain sensation. Often something as simple as changing to a new brand of socks may feel like walking on burning sandpaper.

If hidden medical problems and sensory issues are ruled out, the tantrums or outbursts may stem from a purely behavioral reason. The three major behavioral sources of tantrums, hitting and meltdowns are:

- frustration because the person cannot communicate
- the need for attention
- to escape from a task they do not want to do

Deciphering the correct motivator is important. Once the motivator has been found, a solution can be developed. Otherwise, while is it possible to extinguish an inappropriate behavior, in all likelihood an equally inappropriate behavior that meets the same need will develop. For example, ignoring the behavior is the correct response if the behavior motivator is to seek attention. However, this response would be the worst thing to do if the individual was frustrated because he could not communicate his need for help. Solutions to the behavior could include teaching the child sign language or to use an augmentative communication device. Or teaching the individual socially appropriate ways of saying "no" or expressing his desires.

Keeping a detailed diary will help you figure out the behavior motivation. One nonverbal boy screamed to get his mother to stop at McDonald's because he had learned that it worked. However, he never screamed when his father was driving because he knew dad would not stop.

Frustration with not being able to communicate is a very common problem in nonverbal individuals with ASD; they must have a way to express their needs and wants. If a functional communication system has not been put into place with a child, his only recourse is behavior. I can remember screaming when   I did not want to wear a hat. I had no other way to express my dislike for it, nor to communicate that for me, the hat was disturbing on a sensory level.

Consistency is calming; surprises produce anxiety in most individuals with ASD. They need to know what is coming up next. Sensory processing systems in some of these individuals are so disordered that touch and smell are the only two senses that provide reliable, accurate information to the person's brain. If their visual and auditory systems are giving them jumbled information, they may rely more on touch. This is why some nonverbal people tap things like a blind person navigating with a cane. The neurological feedback this provides is calming to their senses It also explains some of the repetitive behaviors common to individuals with autism. The consistency provided by doing the same thing again and again— and getting the same result—alleviates some of the anxiety associated with the rest of the world being in a constant state of change.

Because of the visual processing problems experienced by many non-verbal individuals with ASD, picture schedules may work poorly with some of them. At one group home, many outbursts and tantrums were avoided by using a touch schedule instead of a picture schedule. Ten minutes before breakfast, they were given a spoon to hold and ten minutes before a shower, they were given a wash cloth. The tangible object communicated what was to happen and the ten-minute period gave their brains time to process the sensory information.

Research is also now showing very clearly that exercise will reduce anxiety and stereotypical behavior. At another group home, a program of vigorous exercise reduced behavior problems.

Some nonverbal teenagers and adults on the spectrum may need medication to alleviate stress and anxiety so that other forms of behavior modification can be used successfully. Often a combination of approaches is best. Sometimes a small dose of conventional medication combined with dietary or other biomedical treatment is more effective than either method used alone.

References

Ankenman, R. 2014. *Hope for the Violently Aggressive Child.* Future Horizons, Arlington, TX.

Aull, E. 2014. *The Parents' Guide to the Medical World of Autism.* Future Horizons, Arlington, TX.

Coleman, R.S. et al. 1976. The effects of fluorescent and incandescent illumination upon repetitive behaviors in autistic children. *Journal of Autism and Developmental Disorders* 6: 157-162.

Hollander, E. et al. 2010. Divalproex sodium vs placebo for the treatment of irritability in children and adolescents with autism spectrum disorders. *Neuropharmacology* 35: 990-998.

Parkin, M. S. et al. 2010. Psychopharmacology of aggressions in children and adolescents with autism: A critical review of efficacy and tolerability. *Journal of Child and Adolescent Psychopharmacology* 18: 157-178.

Strohle, A. et al. 2005. The acute antipanic activity of exercise. *American Journal of Psychiatry* 162: 2376-2378.

Walters, R.G. and W.E. Walters. 1980. Decreasing self-stimulatory behaviors with physical exercise in a group of autistic boys. *Journal of Autism and Developmental Disorders* 10: 379-387.

Whole-Task Teaching for Individuals with Severe Autism

The standard method for teaching a nonverbal person with autism tasks such as dressing or cooking is to provide a picture schedule that shows the steps of the task. This works well for many individuals, but some have difficulty linking the steps together. To learn a simple task such as making a sandwich, they have to see a person demonstrate the *entire* task, from start to finish, with no steps left out. If they do not see how the second slice of bread gets on top of the peanut butter they may not try to perform the individual steps because, as a whole, they do not make sense to the individual. Sandwich-making is easy to teach because when the task is demonstrated, the entire task is observed, and the end product—the sandwich—is concrete and has meaning to the individual.

This idea of "whole-task teaching" is particularly relevant in the area of toilet training. One of the challenges with toilet training individuals on the severe end of the spectrum is that the individual may not know how the urine or feces gets into the toilet. The picture schedule shows the waste in the toilet, but it does not show how it got there. There are often more problems with teaching the person to defecate in the toilet compared to urination. This is because the individual has more likely been able to directly observe how urine comes out of the person and goes into the toilet. This is especially true with boys, but even girls can observe this. It is not as obvious an action—for either sex—when it comes to defecating. If seeing how the waste goes from the person to the toilet is left out of the teaching sequence, these individuals may not know what they have to do.

Furthermore, neurotypicals assume a picture is all that's needed to help the child or adult link the elimination of bodily waste to the place where it should go, i.e., the toilet. But for many individuals that link is too broad a jump and does not "compute" in their brain. Those with severe sensory issues may not feel the sensation of having to urinate or understand how to bear down to defecate. These are intermittent steps that may need to be addressed for a successful toileting program.

Sometimes even demonstrating a whole task via visual teaching is not enough. Many individuals on the severe end of the spectrum have so many visual processing problems that they have to learn tasks by touch. One therapist taught a child how to use a playground slide by "walking" him through the entire task hand-over-hand with no steps left out. To understand how to climb the ladder and go down the slide, the therapist stood behind the child and moved his hands and feet through the entire sequence: climbing the ladder, sitting on the slide, and going down it.

Teaching how a foot is put into a shoe can be done in a similar manner. The therapist, hand-over-hand, guides the individual's hand over the ankle and foot so the person can feel the foot, then feel the inside of the shoe so they can cognitively link how the foot could slide into the shoe. The next step, hand-overhand, is to slip the foot into the shoe in one continuous motion, so the individual experiences the feeling of the foot going into the shoe and makes the cognitive connection through the tactile information being received. Tito, in his book, *How Can I Talk If My Lips Don't Move?* describes learning how to put on a t-shirt. His mother very slowly manipulated the shirt onto him so he could feel his hands going through the sleeves and his head slowly going through the neck opening. If the shirt was put on too rapidly he was not able to process the sensory feedback the material provided and feel the experience.

Individuals on the more severe end of the autism spectrum can be taught to perform different actions, but we must not lose sight of the accompanying sensory issues that can impede their learning. In many cases, these sensory issues are severe and rob the individual of much of the "data feedback" necessary for learning that neurotypicals receive unconsciously. Whole-task, visual, and tactile-based teaching strategies can supply the extra information these individuals need in order to learn.

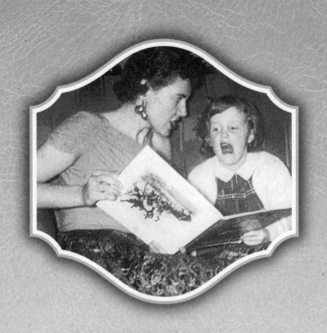

CHAPTER 5

Behavior Issues

Behavior never occurs in a vacuum;
it is the end result of the interaction
between the child and his or her
environment, and that environment
includes the people in it.

B ehavior is one of the most widely discussed topics of all times by parents and professionals within the autism community. Parents want to know how to deal with their child's behaviors at home and in the community. Educators in the classroom find it difficult to manage the behavior outbursts that can accompany autism, and often resort to punitive tactics, which have little or no effect on an autistic child who is having a tantrum due to sensory overload or social misunderstandings. Understanding the source of "bad" behavior and teaching "good" behaviors is a challenge for neurotypical adults who have a different way of thinking and sensing their world than do children with ASD. It requires adults to rethink the way they interact with people with ASD, and most are ill-equipped to do so. Abstract concepts about morality and behavior do not work. The child has to learn by specific examples. When I said something rude about the appearance of a lady at a store, Mother instantly corrected me and explained that commenting on how fat the person is was rude. I had to learn the concept of "rude behavior" by being corrected every time I did a rude behavior. Behavior has to be taught one *specific* example at a time.

Call me old-fashioned, but adults in the world of my youth, the '50s and '60s, believed in a stricter social behavior code than do adults in today's world. For the child with ASD, that was a good thing. Social skills were taught as a matter of course. Behavior rules were straightforward and strictly enforced, another positive strategy well aligned with the autism way of thinking.

Consequences were uniformly imposed and expectations to behave were high. My mother and all the other mothers who lived in our neighborhood attended to children's behaviors, and placed value on teaching their children good manners and appropriate behaviors. To be a functioning member of society, these things were required, not optional, as they seem to be today. Kids today are allowed to do just about anything. The behavior of many five or six-year-olds I've witnessed in stores or other public places is atrocious. The parent stands there, not knowing what to do, eventually giving in to the child's tantrum just to get him quiet.

Today's fast paced, techno-driven world is louder and busier than the world I grew up in. That, in and of itself, creates new challenges for the child with autism, whose sensory systems are usually impaired in one way or another. Our senses are bombarded on a daily basis, and this can render even typical children and adults exhausted by the end of the day. Imagine the effect it has on the sensory-sensitive systems of the child with autism, especially those with hyper-acute senses. They enter the world with a set of physical challenges that severely impair their ability to tolerate life, let alone learn within conventional environments. They have so much farther to go to be ready to learn than I did growing up in my time.

When figuring out how to handle behavior problems, one has to ask: Is it a *sensory* problem or a *behavior* problem? Accommodations are usually needed to help a child handle problems with sensory oversensitivity. Punishing sensory problems will just make the child's behavior *worse*. Sometimes behavior problems occur when an individual with ASD becomes frustrated due to slower mental processing, which in turn makes a quick response difficult. In kindergarten, I threw a huge tantrum because the teacher did not give me enough time to explain the mistakes I had made on an assignment. The task was to mark pictures of things that began with the letter B. I was marked wrong for marking a picture of a suitcase with the letter B. In our house, suitcases were called "bags."

Behavior never occurs in a vacuum; it is the end result of the interaction between the child and his or her environment, and that environment includes the people in it. To bring about positive change in the behavior of the child with ASD, adults need to first adjust their own behaviors. In the television series, Supernanny, Jo Frost makes such remarkable changes in the behavior of kids because she first helps parents get control of their own behaviors and learn basic behavior techniques. That's a valuable lesson for every parent, educator, or service provider, to take to heart. The behavior, good or bad, of a child with ASD, largely depends on you and your behavior. If you want to change the behavior of the child, first look at your own. You might be surprised by what you see.

In solving behavioral problems, parents and teachers tend to overgeneralize. They will ask me how I deal with a behavioral problem at school. To develop an effective solution requires much more detailed information, such as age, description of the behavior, and level of verbal skills. After asking many questions, I can determine that one child is going into sensory overload and another child is behaving badly because he is being forced to do the same "baby math" over and over, and he is bored. Therefore, one child needs a more challenging math book, and the other may need to get away from the noise in the cafeteria.

The way I see it, many parents and teachers do not hold high enough expectations for good behavior from these individuals, nor do they hold them responsible for their behaviors.

Disability versus Just Bad Behaviors

During my travels, I have observed that many children on the autism spectrum need more discipline. Many parents and teachers seem confused about the cause of some of the behaviors that surface from within their kids. Is it just bad behavior or is the problem behavior caused by the person's disability?

Teachers and parents need to differentiate between a troublesome behavior caused by sensory problems and just plain bad behavior. This is especially true for highly verbal autistic and Asperger's children. The way I see it, many parents and teachers do not hold high enough expectations for good behavior from these individuals, nor do they hold them responsible for their behaviors. My being raised during the 1950s probably was an advantage. Life was much more structured then. I was expected to behave when my family sat down for dinner. It was quiet at the house during dinner so there were no problems with sensory overload. Today, in the average household, dinner can be noisy, chaotic, and stressful for a child on the spectrum. Music is playing or the TV is on, or siblings are all talking or yelling at one time. To my mother's credit, she was also a good detective about what environments caused me stress. She recognized that large, noisy crowds or too much noise and commotion in general was more than my nervous system could handle. When I had a tantrum, she understood why.

Bad behaviors should have consequences, and parents need to understand that applying consequences in a consistent manner will make gains in changing these behaviors. I behaved well at the dining room table because there were consequences: I lost TV privileges for one night if I misbehaved at the table. Other misbehaving, such as swearing or laughing at a fat lady, had consequences. Mother knew how to make consequences meaningful, too. She chose those things that were important to me, such as my privileges.

I was always testing the limits, as most children will. Parents should not think that because their child has autism or Asperger's this will not happen. Mother made sure there was consistent discipline at home, and between home and school. She, my nanny, and my teacher worked together. There was no way I could manipulate one against the other. The table on the following page shows some examples of "just bad behavior" and some of the more common behavior problems caused by either high-functioning autism or Asperger's Syndrome. Many of these examples came directly from parents and teachers I've met at workshops and conferences. Bad behavior needs discipline. But parents must never punish a child with autism for acting out, or having a tantrum, when it is caused by sensory overload or some other part of autism, such as not comprehending what is expected of him or her, or never being taught appropriate social skills. If you know your child well, and understand how the various sensory and social systems are affected by autism, you'll know when your child's behavior is "just plain bad" and when it's a manifestation of his or her autism.

BAD BEHAVIOR that should be corrected. Autism, ASD or Asperger's Syndrome is NOT an excuse

- Sloppy table manners
- Dressing like a slob; poor grooming
- Being rude to a teacher, a parent, another adult, or a peer
- Swearing
- Laughing inappropriately at people (e.g., at a fat lady, someone in a wheelchair)
- Inappropriate sexual behavior in public
- Manipulating adults by throwing fits at home, school or in the community
- Stealing a toy and then lying about it
- Cheating at a card game or during a sports activity

Behavior Problems caused by Autism, ASD, or Asperger's Syndrome. ACCOMMODATIONS may be required

- Screaming when the fire alarm rings because it hurts his ears
- Tantruming in a large, busy supermarket/mall/recreation area due to sensory overload; more likely to occur when the child is tired
- Removing clothes/excessive scratching/itching: cannot tolerate feel of certain fabrics, seams, fibers against skin
- Hyperactivity and agitation under fluorescent lighting
- Sloppy handwriting: often due to poor fine-motor skills. (Allow child to use typewriter or computer instead.)
- Difficulties with multi-tasking due to the brain's slower processing speed

- Problems with following long strings of verbal instructions. Written instructions may be required.
- Problems with multi-tasking
- Need breaks to calm down

Providing a soft object for the client to attack seems to calm the client down, whereas forceful restraint makes the client more angry or scared.

My Experience with Teasing and Bullying

In elementary school, I had friends because the other children enjoyed doing craft projects with me. I was good at making things that the other children were interested in, projects such as kites or tree houses. I had friends through shared interests. Another reason why I had a good elementary school experience without bullying is that my third-grade teacher, Mrs. Dietsch, explained to the other children that I had a disability that was not visible like crutches or a wheelchair. She encouraged the other children to help me learn social rules. Today, this approach is called "peer-mediated intervention." My big bullying problems happened in high school.

In high school, teenagers become purely social beings. Being good at crafts or science projects did not score any points in the social scene. The children's rhyme says, "Sticks and stones will break your bones, but words will never hurt you." That is not true; words hurt a lot.

At first, my response to teasing was anger. I got kicked out of a large girl's school for throwing a book at a girl who called me a "retard." In ninth grade, I went to a small boarding school for gifted but troubled students. Within the first week, the teasing started. They called me "bones" because

I was skinny, and "tape recorder." I responded with fists. After a major fistfight in the cafeteria, I had horseback riding privileges revoked. Since I really wanted to ride the horses, I stopped fighting. The consequences for fist fighting had an impact on me. I then developed friendships through shared interests in horseback riding and model rockets.

However, the strong emotions I felt did not simply go away. I had to find an outlet for these emotions because they could not just be shut off. So, I started crying when I was teased. Even today, I defuse anger by crying. Angry outbursts would not be tolerated at work, but if I have to cry, I can find a private place.

When I went off to college at Franklin Pierce College in New Hampshire, there were many good teachers who helped me. However, teasing was still a problem. They called me "buzzard woman." The turning point came, and the teasing stopped, when the other students found out that I had talents and useful skills that interested them. I became involved in the school talent show, working many hours making scenery and acting in some of the skits. I made a sign for the Old Palace Theatre, covered with silver glitter, with orange and green lettering. I also sang some funny songs in a screeching voice.

Until a person participates in activities that are shared with other people, the bullying will continue. I strongly recommend that students with autism/AS get involved in special interest clubs in some of the areas they naturally excel at such as computers, art, math, karate, etc. Some other good activities are scouting, showing animals in 4-H or Future Farmers of America, and Maker Community Groups. Maker Community Groups do cool things with three-dimensional printers. These clubs will help provide a refuge from teasing and improve the person's self-esteem. Being with people who share your interests makes socializing easier.

As I have said many times before, talents need to be developed. Parents and teachers need to work on expanding the child's range of interests into areas that can be shared with other students. For example, the student with autism may have good art skills, but all he draws are doorknobs. Skills such as drawing need to be broadened. A good first step may be to enroll the student in an art class where drawing other subjects is required. I can remember when I took a pencil sketching class and had to spend the entire two hour class drawing my own shoe. At college, the other students didn't become interested in my artistic talents until I made scenery for the school show. We all shared a common goal—the show—and I became part of their "group."

While I made scenery for some of my high school plays, the young teenagers were too hyper-social to appreciate my abilities. Some gifted autistic or Asperger's students may need to be removed from this hyper-social high school scene. Enroll them in a university or community college course where they can be with their intellectual peers. College students are a bit more mature and they recognize and appreciate talents and don't tease as much. In high school, I dropped out of the teenage social scene because it was too hard for me to deal with. It was not until the college talent show that I was able to participate again.

References and Additional Readings

Charlop, M.H. et al. (2018) Want to play? Peer medicated intervention of young children with autism spectrum disorder, In: Play and Social Skills for Children with Autism Spectrum Disorder, *Evidence Based Practices in Behavioral Health*, Springer, pp. 107-127.

Daniel, L.S. et al. (2010) What boys with autism have to say about establishing and maintaining friendships, *Focus on Autism and Other Developmental Disabilities*, 25:220-229.

Grandin, T. (2018) *Calling All Minds: How to Think and Create Like an Inventor*, Penguin Random House, New York NY.

Hong, E.R. et al. (2015) Addressing bullying of students with autism: Suggestions for parents and educators, *Intervention in School and Clinic*, 50:157-162.

Koenig, K.P. et al. (2017) Characterization and utilization of preferred special interests: A survey of adults on the autism spectrum, *Occupational Therapy and Mental Health*, 33:129-140.

Pierce, K. and Schreibman, L. (1995) Increasing complex social behavior in children with autism: Effects of peer implemented pivotal response training, *Journal of Applied Behavior Analysis*, 28:285-295.

Watkins, L. et al. (2015) Review of peer mediated social interaction for students with autism in inclusive settings, *Journal of Autism and Developmental Disorders*, 45:1070-1083.

The anger and resentment many people with AS feel is understandable and justified. What is not, however, is rude "acting-out behavior" in response to these feelings.

Rudeness is Inexcusable

Recently I went to a large autism meeting here in the US and was appalled at the rude behavior exhibited by a few adult individuals with Asperger's Syndrome (AS) who were also attending. One of them walked up to me and said, "Who the f— are you?" He also interrupted two major sessions at the conference because he adamantly opposed the notion of finding a cure for autism. Later that day, this same individual ran a panel discussion where individuals with AS talked about their lives. During this session, his manners and behavior were polite and perfect, demonstrating he was capable of behaving properly when he wanted to.

What was most distressing to me was that these individuals felt that because they had Asperger's, the people around them should accept their rude behavior—that their "disability" made them somehow exempt from the social standards we all live by. Like it or not, social boundaries exist that we are expected to conform to, whether we're members of a "minority" population or mainstream American society. To be members of a group, we must all learn the rules and act in socially appropriate ways.

People with autism and AS may find this more difficult to do, but being on the spectrum is not an exemption from doing so.

I wasn't entirely opposed to some of the viewpoints these individuals with AS shared with other conference attendees, but I couldn't help but think how much more effective they could have been in the delivery of their message so that other people at the conference would be willing to listen and consider what they had to say. Rude behavior has consequences, and in most cases, they are negative. In general, rude or overt anti-social behavior:

- is an instant turn-off; most people dislike those who are rude.
- makes people uncomfortable, uneasy.
- closes down channels of communication.
- results in people forming quick negative opinions about you, whether or not they are valid or based on fact.
- alienates you from others; it reduces the chance of further contact.
- is seen as individual weakness, as an inability of a person to be "in control" of his or her emotions.

Those of us with autism/AS live in a society that can be grossly ignorant of our needs, of the day-by-day difficulty we face in trying to "fit" into a world that is often harsh, stressful, and grating on our neurology. The anger and resentment many people with AS feel is understandable and justified. What is not, however,

is rude "acting-out behavior" in response to these feelings, and calling that behavior acceptable in the name of autism.

The autism and the neurotypical cultures remain divided, yet that gap is slowly closing through education, awareness, and experiences. It happens one person at a time, and we each play a role in how quickly we close the gap. When individuals with AS tout a rigid belief that they should be allowed to act in any way they choose, exempt from the social rules that call for respect for our fellow man, they widen the chasm that still exists. It perpetuates a we-versus-them mentality: "You are wrong; we are right." It also perpetuates the very negative stereotypes some of us on the spectrum work to overturn: that people with AS are stubborn, resistant to change, and unwilling to compromise. While these may be characteristics of autism spectrum disorders, to put forth the notion that these are immutable, unchangeable personality traits only further supports the "inability" of people on the spectrum.

The best way to teach the child is to use "teachable" moments. When a child makes a social mistake, do not scream "NO." Instead, give instruction. For example, if a child reaches across the dining room table for the food, tell him to ask his mother or sister to pass it.

If a child pushes in line at the movie theater, tell him, "You have to wait your turn for a ticket." If he makes a rude comment about a person at the grocery store, pull him aside and say, "It is rude to discuss other people's appearance in public." The key is to calmly give instruction and to not start screaming at the child.

I have talked to many parents who have told me their child is good at drawing or some other skill but keeps destroying their work because it has some minor imperfection.

The Need to Be Perfect

S ome individuals on the autism spectrum who are good at drawing or other skills will often destroy excellent work because it is not absolutely perfect. Sean Barron, a well-known individual on the spectrum, described how he destroyed a beautiful airplane he had made—one that had taken many, many hours to create—because it had one small flaw. In his mind, if the plane was not perfect, it had no value. Other individuals will delete good artwork from their computer because they think it is inferior. Some children will tear up pages of homework because of one small spelling correction or because too much erasing makes the page look messy.

Other individuals on the autism spectrum conceal their ability. One mother discovered that her nonverbal son, who, to her knowledge, could not read, was typing words such as "depression" into Google. This is very different than a child or adult typing a memorized cartoon character's name into YouTube so he can watch videos. Memorizing a cartoon character's name requires no reading skills, but typing words such as "depression" or "Iraq" may indicate an individual has some hidden reading skills. I told his mother to download the computer's cache memory to look at her son's search history to determine if he was possibly reading about either "Iraq" or "depression." Neither of these words were part of the boy's schoolwork;

however, he was exposed to them by the people around him. By looking at his search history, the mother could determine if her son might be concealing his reading ability.

Even Experts Are Not Perfect

People with autism and Asperger's Syndrome tend towards black-and white thinking. They see themselves and the world around them in polar opposites, and this tendency feeds their need to be perfect. Even the tiniest mistakes and mishaps can feel like monumental failures to them, creating high levels of anxiety when their efforts or the events around them do not measure up to this all-or-nothing scale.

I have talked to many parents who have told me their child is good at drawing or some other skill but keeps destroying their work because it has some minor imperfection. It is important for parents to teach a child, in concrete ways, that 1) skills exist on a continuum and 2) there are different levels of quality required for different levels of work. To start, explain to the child that even the greatest experts in a field may have imperfections in their work. For example, being a photographer for *National Geographic* requires a person to be the very best. A photographer for *Time* or *Newsweek* has to be good, but not as good as a photographer for *National Geographic*. In other words, there are different levels of quality for photography work. They could be listed like this:

- Expert photographer—Works at *National Geographic*
- Very good photographer—Works at *New York Times, Newsweek*, or *Wall Street Journal*
- Good photographer—Works doing local weddings, portraits, or local commercial photography

- Good amateur—Takes nice scenic vacation pictures
- Snapshot taker—takes snapshots of average quality
- Terrible photographer—Takes totally bad pictures: cuts off heads, overexposes film, pictures are blurred, or makes other immediately obvious mistakes.

As the quality categories of the photos decline, the pictures will contain more and more mistakes. It is equally important that an individual see concrete examples of the best AND the worst to develop perspective. If you look hard enough, it is even possible to find mistakes in photos in *National Geographic* magazines; not all their photos are absolutely perfect. A person can have a good career in photography if his pictures are in categories 1, 2, or 3.

Giving individuals concrete, visual representations of the different levels of photography can help them better understand the continuum of skills. A mentor or teacher can reinforce these ideas, showing the individual many examples of photos for each category and even helping the individual sort photos into the different categories. The individual can then strive for *National Geographic* or *Time Magazine* quality instead of perfection.

When the student looks at one of his own photos, he can be reinforced to ask himself, "Is this good enough for categories 1, 2, or 3?" instead of getting angry and destroying his work because it is not perfect.

When I was getting started, I had the opposite problem. I sometimes did sloppy work on tasks that did not interest me.

In my twenties, I did a very sloppy job making copies of sales brochures. A good way to instruct me would have been to show me an example of a quality copy job and contrast that with an example of a poor copy job, while explaining what makes one good and the other bad. For instance, crooked copies are not acceptable. Copies missing any pages are not acceptable. The quality of work can be measured along a range from excellent (though not totally perfect) to terrible. These categories are similar to the thermometer scales used with individuals with autism/AS to teach different levels of emotions.

A quality scale can be used in many different applications, from writing to computer programming. For writing, the categories could range from major literary works to local newspaper writing to poor school papers. Make sure students see specific examples of each category.

Teach your child love and kindness in a concrete manner, with very specific examples.

Autism & Religion: Teach Goodness

Many parents share with me their desire to educate their child with autism or Asperger's about the religion practiced by the rest of their family. Some wonder if their child is capable of understanding the concept of God, or a higher power, of being spiritual, or even understanding the basic messages of the Bible or other religious texts.

I have learned, over the years, that there is a whole upper layer of abstract thought mixed with emotion that I do not have. Thoughts and emotions are separated in my mind; they don't intermingle and affect one another. Thinking is concrete—it happens in pictures in my mind. Therefore, for me, inspirational matters had no meaning, except for the very concrete aspects of them taught to me.

I had a proper religious upbringing, though. My family attended the Episcopalian church every Sunday. These weekly outings held little value for me, and I was not interested in what went on. The scratchy petticoats I had to wear to church were awful; in fact, the worst thing about church was the Sunday-best clothes. Sunday school was boring to me and I usually spent the entire class filling in the Os and Ps in the church program.

However, sitting still through an activity that was boring was good discipline. It taught me that sometimes I had to participate in activities that were boring because that is what the rest of the family wanted to do. Often, one has to do activities that other people want to do. This is a more abstract version of learning how to take turns.

Concrete teachings were what I understood. For instance, our Christmas service made a lasting impression on me that I retain to this day. Each Christmas, every child in the congregation had to take one of their good toys and give it to a poor child. One year, I offered my yo-yo and Mother told me that I had to give a better present. At the Christmas service, the minister stood next to the manger, full of donated toys, and said, "It is better to give than to receive." This kind of concrete learning I understood.

The autistic/Asperger's mind tends to dwell on negatives, and this is something parents and professionals should be aware of and find ways to counteract. It is beneficial for a young autistic or Asperger's child to be schooled with positive teachings. One way to do this is through religious training. Helping a child understand what to do, in concrete ways, demonstrating actions that are giving and positive and helpful to others, can counterbalance this tendency toward negative thinking. If a child asks about something negative, for instance, like stoning as it's mentioned in the Bible, I would recommend parents telling the child that in modern times, most people no longer do that. Keep it concrete and simple.

A nice, positive approach for a Christian upbringing would be to give a child one of the WWJD—"What Would Jesus Do?" necklaces or key chains. Then teach the child concrete examples of what Jesus did, or would do, in various situations.

For instance, Jesus would not cheat at games. He would not lie, or steal another child's toys. When I was little, I stole a toy fire engine from another child and Mother made me give it back.

Moral upbringing must be concrete. A good person is considerate of others. One example I remember from my childhood was being told, by a very sleepy mother, that asking her to open a stuck glue bottle while she was sleeping was not being considerate. Fair play and good sportsmanship are important to teach. Jesus would play fairly and would not be a poor loser. He would not scream and rant if he lost a game. It is unfortunate that in our society today, so many sports heroes behave badly on television and there are no consequences for their actions. It teaches a wrong moral lesson for a child with autism or Asperger's (or any child) to see a famous basketball player not being punished for kicking a TV camera man. If a child views things like this, it is important that a parent tell the child that Jesus would never do that.

Teach your child love and kindness in a concrete manner, with very specific examples. For instance, an example of kindness would be bringing flowers to an elderly lady in a nursing home. There are hundreds of ways parents can share the real essence of their faith with their child with autism or Asperger's, through daily demonstrations of the goodness that is at the foundation of their religion. This is more important, and will help the child in the future more than will learning to recite passages of text, or trying to teach them higher-level concepts that they will have difficulty understanding.

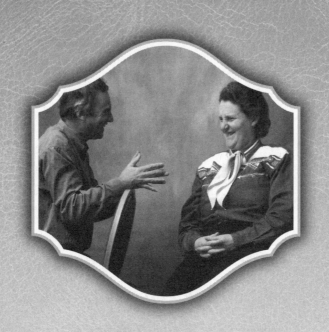

CHAPTER 6

Social Functioning

The way I see it, a huge mistake many teachers and parents make is to try to make people with autism or Asperger's into something they are not—turn the geeky nerd into an ungeek, for instance.

T here are hundreds of papers in the scientific literature about problems people on the autism spectrum have with social thinking and Theory of Mind (ToM). Theory of Mind is the ability to understand what other people may be thinking. In its most elementary form, it's the ability to understand that different people have different thoughts. Involved within ToM is perspective taking, being able to think about and understand an event or a situation "through the eyes of another." These are all social thinking skills that develop without formal instruction in neurotypical individuals, starting at a very early age. These are also skills that most people, including educators, assume exist in all people, to a greater or lesser degree of development. This is not the case within the autism population.

Without a fully functioning social thinking system, individuals with higher functioning autism or Asperger's Syndrome (HFA/AS) stumble along through academic and social situations, missing valuable bits of verbal nuance or nonverbal body messages that are woven into typical conversation. The impairment can be pervasive, even among those with higher intelligence. For instance, a middle school child who can wax eloquent about the anatomical differences among different varieties of alligators may not understand the simple social convention of turning his body towards his conversational partner to indicate interest in what he has to say. In the world of higher functioning autism, neither verbal ability nor IQ is an indication of equivalent social aptitude and social thinking/reasoning skills. The most basic of social skills may be missing.

Individuals on the more severe end of the spectrum have difficulty with the elementary levels of ToM and perspective taking. I have always been able to pass a simple Theory of Mind test. An example of such a test would go like this. I am in a room with Jim and Bob. Bob puts a candy bar in a box and Jim leaves the room. While Jim is out of the room, Bob moves the candy bar from the box to a desk drawer. When Jim returns, I know that he thinks the candy bar is still in the box. If I had impaired Theory of Mind, I would think that Jim also knows the candy bar was moved to the desk drawer, because I saw him move the candy bar, and if I know it, so does everyone else.

I process this test purely with my photo-realistic visual thinking. I picture Jim outside with the door closed; he could not possibly see the candy bar being moved. When I was given a more complex Theory of Mind test, I did poorly because it required remembering a sequence of several events involving children and an ice cream truck. Plus, the test was presented verbally, which made remembering it even more difficult for my visual thinking mind. My ability to remember spoken word sequence is absolutely terrible. When I ask for directions, I have to write them down to remember the sequence. With the second ToM test, my problem was not in understanding another person's viewpoint, it was with my sequencing skills. Written instructions are best for me, as they are for a majority of children and adults with ASD.

Visual Theory of Mind

My mother taught me when I was very young—again, by using visual examples—the importance of understanding how another person feels. When I was about eight, I ate with my mouth open and Mother kept telling me to keep it closed when I was chewing my food. She kept telling me to close my mouth, but I still chewed with it open because it made no sense to me why it was important. Then one day I came home from school and I told mother that watching Billy eat with his mouth open made me gag, that it looked like the inside of a garbage truck. Mother quietly replied, "Your mouth looks like the inside of a garbage truck when it is open and it makes me want to gag." Now I understood that mother was experiencing the same response that I had experienced when I saw Billy chew with his mouth open. To understand how another person felt in the situation, I had to experience myself what the other child was experiencing. For children who are less visual learners and respond well to verbal language, it may work to tell them that the rule is to chew with their mouth closed.

Avoid Being Abstract

Conversely, it is also difficult for people who think abstractly to understand situations where non-abstract thinking is necessary. This can present career opportunities for people with ASD. In my job designing livestock facilities, nothing is abstract. Abstract thinking is not required to design and build things. This is why I like my career so much. I get a great sense of accomplishment improving the conditions for animals, and now half the cattle in the U.S. and Canada are handled in equipment I have designed. I can see tangible results of my work; it is not abstract. I also get great satisfaction when I can help a parent or teacher solve a problem with a child. When parents tell me that one of my books helped them understand their child and enabled them to work with him more effectively, it makes me really happy.

To be an effective teacher with a child with HFA/AS, explain the rules of living in a non-abstract manner. Do not say to a child, "Well, you have to be good because it is the right thing to do." The words "good" and "right" are much too abstract for the concrete thinking mind of the spectrum child. Instead be specific and say, "You should take turns playing the game because, if another child was playing, you would want him to give you a turn to play." Another concrete example would be something like, "Do not steal the other child's toys because you would not like it if he took your things." Teach the Golden Rule, one specific example at a time.

I Am What I Do

Another reason having a good career is so important to me is that I am what I do instead of what I feel. For me, emotional complexity is replaced with intellectual complexity. My greatest satisfaction in life comes from doing things. My best social interactions always involved activities with others with whom I shared a common interest, such as building things or animal behavior. Many of my friends are either in animal behavior, involved with building projects, or work on the animal welfare issue. I also have lots of good friends in the autism community. My career gives my life meaning. This is the way many "techies" feel. To me, intellectual reason and knowledge are extremely valuable. This is why I was so upset ten years ago when the library at our university was flooded. I was upset about books and knowledge being destroyed.

Over the several decades I have been involved with the autism/ Asperger's community, I have learned that some individuals on the spectrum share my way of relating to life and the world, and others do not. There are individuals with HFA/ AS who have a few more social emotional circuits connected in their brain, and for them, feelings and emotional connection with others is a bigger part of their functioning. This also, however, produces a greater level of frustration in many parts of their lives, such as friendships and dating. The life of celibacy that I lead would not be right for them. This spectrum of emotional differences in individuals with HFA/ AS became even more illuminated for me while working with Sean Barron on our 2005 book, *Unwritten Rules of Social Relationships*. It was a real eye opener for me to learn that two successful adults with AS can relate to the world so differently, and see where we were almost the same in many ways, and where we were so different. While I am really happy that at that time Sean had a girlfriend and a good romantic relationship in his life, that is not a choice that would work for me. Romantic relationships are too abstract for my way of thinking. An article about our differences is included in this chapter.

Sensory-Based Empathy

I can empathize through my senses rather than in a more emotional abstract manner. When I see cattle in the mud, I can empathize with how cold and miserable they feel. One of the things I can empathize with is physical hardship. When the home mortgage mess in 2007 caused many people to lose their homes, it made me angry. The shoeshine lady at the Denver airport lost her home after taking out an adjustable rate mortgage that she did not understand, and then couldn't meet the escalated payments. When business takes advantage of the poor and less educated of our society, it makes me mad.

People on the spectrum often have a strong sense of social justice. This sense is probably on a separate brain current from the circuits that are responsible for emotional relatedness between people. This sense of social justice is within me, too. Every time I read another article in the newspaper about people losing their homes due to unethical business practices, it makes me furious.

When I took psychology classes in college, I studied Maslow's Pyramid of Needs. At the bottom are food, shelter, and safety, and at the top are the abstract ideals of self-actualization, a concept that remains nebulous to me. I am much more concerned about the bottom of the pyramid, those things that affect people's lives on a concrete level, than I am interested in ideology. I understand concrete results. The only ideology that interests me is that which results in real, tangible improvements happening on the ground level. In the autism/Asperger's world, that would be an ideology that produces a good outcome for a child. A nonverbal child should have the opportunities to grow up and have a meaningful life in a group home and possibly hold a job, depending on their level of functioning. People on the higher end of the spectrum should be able to live independently, work, and contribute to society as their own interests and viewpoints dictate. For the really smart Asperger's individuals, a college education and a career is a reasonable goal.

Some of the HFA/AS individuals who feel emotional connectedness, who pursue not just social but romantic relationships, may find success in dating or marrying another person who shares their traits. Socialization through a shared interest, such as a science fiction or history club, are often where the first dates occur. I have talked to many neurotypical spouses who do not understand a husband who is Asperger's. They are concerned about his lack of social emotional relatedness. I explain to them that social skills can be learned like acting in a play. The brain circuits may not be hooked up for emotional relatedness, but he can be a good provider, a good parent, and very loyal. These individuals often possess many good traits, such as honesty, dedication, steadfastness, and a sense of social justice, that can be good in a marriage.

I Am a Nerd

The way I see it, a huge mistake many teachers and parents make is to try to make people with autism or Asperger's into something they are not—turn the geeky nerd into an ungeek, for instance. That just won't work. Teaching them to be socially functional is a worthy goal and one not to be overlooked. However, it would be in everybody's best interest to remember that the world is made up of all sorts of individuals, and that geeks, nerds, and people with mild Asperger's are often one and the same thing. I can learn social rules, but I will never have the undercurrent of social emotional relatedness that exists in some people. The neural circuits that connect those parts of the brain just aren't hard-wired in me.

I have heard sad stories where a mother took her teenager out of computer classes that he truly enjoyed to place him in situations to make him more social. That was a totally wrong thing to do for two reasons. First, it robs him of the opportunity to develop a talent and interest that could lead to future employment. Second, the teen's social experiences are going to more naturally unfold and progress with the other computer students'— those with whom he has shared interests. The happy geeks excel at their jobs and get to work in Silicon Valley where they are appreciated for their brains. The unhappy geeks end up without activities to keep them intellectually stimulated, and instead, are forced into uncomfortable social situations that, more often than not, fail to achieve the goal of making them more social. The people in the world who think that social connectedness is the ultimate goal of life forget that telephones, social networking websites, text messaging, and all the other electronic vehicles that fuel their passion to socialize are made by people with some degree of autism. Geeks swoon over the new technology they create; social addicts swoon by communicating with the technology and showing it off as a status symbol. Is one "better" than the other? I think not.

Dr. Nancy Minshew did a functional MRI brain scan on me that indicated that I was innately more interested in looking at videos of things than videos of people. When I did the scan, I had no idea of its purpose. A series of short video clips of people and things such as bridges, buildings, and fruit were shown. I immediately noticed that the videos were old and scratchy and looked like they came from the 1970s. This triggered my mind into problem-solving mode to figure out where the researchers had gotten these old tapes. The pictures of things provided more clues to the origin of the videos than the pictures of people. When the things flashed on the screen, I looked for cars because I wanted to know how old the videos were. My brain reacted by giving more neural activity to pictures of things than people.

There is no right or wrong in the interests and ways of being among individuals with HFA/AS—provided they can function reasonably well within society. If they cannot, further social learning is clearly needed.

When all else is relatively equal, the way I see it, parents and educators should respect the innate interests of the child and nurture their expression. Not everyone in the world is highly social, and that's a good thing. It's the same within the autism spectrum. In another case I learned about, a boy with more severe autism was a great artist. His mother was so upset that he would never marry (her dream for her son), she was hesitant to help him develop his artistic ability. For this kid, art was his life. Fortunately, she was persuaded to start a business selling her son's art. He is content to draw all day, and this gives his life meaning.

The autism/Asperger's spectrum is broad. Many individuals are blessed with a unique ability while others do not have any special skills. But each individual, no matter what level of skills or IQ or social abilities, can become a contributing member of the community. This is what will give meaning to their lives. Our goal, therefore, is not to make these individuals find meaning in our lives, but for us to help individuals with autism/Asperger's find meaning in their own.

Insights into Autistic
Social Problems

An interesting study by Dr. Ami Klin and associates at the Yale Child Study Center is helping to explain some of the social problems in people with autism. Both normal and autistic adults were fitted with a device that tracked their eye movements, allowing the researchers to determine what the person was looking at. Subjects wearing the eye tracking device were shown digitized clips of *Who's Afraid of Virginia Wolf,* a movie that contains a high number of instances of social interaction between people in a living room setting. (It is the kind of movie I find boring, because of its social nature.)

The first finding was that autistic subjects fixate on the mouths of people instead of on their eyes. I think one of the reasons they do this is because of their problems hearing auditory detail. I have problems hearing hard consonant sounds. If somebody says "brook" I know the word is not "crook" if it is spoken in the context of a picnic. Looking at the mouth of the person talking makes hearing the correct word easier. I find that when I am in a noisy room, hearing is more difficult if I look at a person's eyes. I tend to point my good ear towards the person, in order to hear better.

Amy Klin's study also showed that a normal person's gaze rapidly switched back and forth between the eyes of the two people conversing in the movie. This happened with less frequency in a person with autism. In one particular test, the subjects viewed three people conversing. The autistic person's gaze switched only once while the normal subject's gaze moved at least six times among the three people on the screen. This can be explained by attention-shifting delays that are often present in autism. Research conducted by Eric Courchesne, in San Diego, has shown that autistics take much longer to shift attention between two different stimuli than do their normal counterparts. The inability to shift attention quickly may explain some of the social deficits that develop within this population. Even if a person with autism was more aware of social cues that go on between people, their inability to quickly shift focus would prevent them from catching these short, silent messages that people frequently use to communicate nonverbally.

Processing the meaning of eye movements requires many rapid attention shifts. This may partially explain why people with autism may not even be aware of subtle eye movements that often occur during conversations. I did not know that people communicated with their eye movements until I read it in a book, in my early fifties. All my life I existed unaware of this part of communication. As a child, I understood that if a person's head was pointed towards me, they could see me. But I did not notice smaller eye movements. Many adults with au-

tism have commented that they finally discovered, at a later age, that normal people have a language of their eyes; however, they could never understand it. Not being able to rapidly shift attention may be the reason why.

To help people with autism better participate in conversation, people can slow down their speech, talk their thoughts out loud in more detail, instead of using nonverbal eye and body language, and check for comprehension by the person with autism, repeating things if needed.

Learning Social Rules

C hildren and adults on the autism spectrum are concrete, literal thinkers. Ideas that can't be understood through logic or that involve emotions and social relationships are difficult for us to grasp, and even more difficult to incorporate into our daily lives. When I was in high school, figuring out the social rules was a major challenge. It was not easy to notice similarities in people's social actions and responses because they were often inconsistent from person to person and situation to situation. Over time, I observed that some rules could be broken with minor consequences and other rules, when broken, had serious consequences. It perplexed me that other kids seemed to know which rules they could bend and break and which rules must never be broken. They had a flexibility of thinking that I did not have. I knew I had to learn these rules if I wanted to function in social situations. If I had to learn them, they somehow had to be meaningful to me, to make sense to me within my own way of thinking and viewing the world. I started observing others as would a scientist and discovered I could group the rules into an organizational format to which I could relate: into major and minor categories. By the time I was a senior in high school, I had a system for categorizing some of the social rules of life. I still use the same system today.

I developed four rule categories: 1) Really Bad Things; 2) Courtesy Rules; 3) Illegal But Not Bad; and 4) Sins of the System.

Really Bad Things

I reasoned that in order to maintain a civilized society, there must be prohibitions against doing really bad things such as murder, arson, rape, stealing, looting, and injuring other people. If really bad things are not controlled, a civilized society where we have jobs, food in the stores, and electricity cannot exist.

The prohibition against really bad things is universal in all civilized societies. Children need to be taught that cheating—in all forms, not just on tests—is bad. Learning to "play fair" will help a child grow into an adult who will not commit really bad things. The child can be taught the concept of playing fair with many specific examples.

Courtesy Rules

All civilized societies have courtesy rules, such as saying "please" and "thank you." These rules are important because they help prevent anger that can escalate into really bad things. Different societies have different courtesy rules, but they all serve the same function. In most countries, some common courtesy rules are: standing and waiting your turn in a line, good table manners, being neat and clean, giving up your seat on a bus to an elderly person, or raising your hand and waiting for the teacher to point to you before speaking in class.

Illegal But Not Bad

These rules can sometimes be broken depending upon the circumstance. Rules in this category vary greatly from one society to another and how an individual views these rules will be influenced by his or her own set of moral and personal beliefs. Be careful though: consequences for breaking some are minor; for others, there may be a fine. Included in this category is slight speeding in cars. One rule I often recommend breaking is the age requirement for attending a community college. I tell parents to sign up the child so he can escape being teased in high school. However, the parent must impress upon the child that this is a grown-up privilege and he must obey all the courtesy rules. An example of a rule that would not fall in this category would be running a red light. Doing this carries the possibility of injuring or killing someone, which is a Really Bad Thing.

Sins of the System

These are rules that must never be broken, although they may seem to have little or no basis in logic. They must simply be accepted within our country and our culture. For instance, a small sexual transgression that would result in your name being added to a sex-offender list in the U.S. may have little or no consequence in another country. In the U.S., the four major sins of the system are sexual transgressions, drug offenses, making fake IDs, and playing with explosives. Parents have reported to me that their teenager has looked at porn. First of all, he must be made aware of the laws. Forced sex (rape), all sex with underage girls, or looking at child porn has the penalty of prison and being placed on the sex offender list.

In a post-September 11th world, pranks that used to be considered kids being naughty are now being prosecuted as serious crimes. Never commit a "sin of the system" because the penalties are usually very severe.

This method of categorizing social rules has worked well for me. However, each person with autism may need different rule categories that make sense for him or her. The number of sins of the system is increasing. NEVER make threats online to harm or kill people. Threats are NEVER a joke. You can go to jail.

My emotions are all in the present. I can be angry but I get over it quickly.

Emotional Differences Among Individuals with Autism or Asperger's

I gained some valuable insight into both myself and others on the autism spectrum when I worked with Sean Barron on our book, *Unwritten Rules of Social Relationships: Decoding Social Mysteries Through the Unique Perspectives of Autism*. There were areas where Sean and I shared similar emotions and other areas where emotional relatedness was experienced almost opposite one another. We both are independent, well-functioning adults, with varied interests and social relationships, yet our socialemotional development took very different paths.

We were similar in two main areas: rigid, black-and-white thinking and singular obsessions. In elementary school, Sean obsessed over the exact angle of parked school busses. My obsession was collecting election and wrestling posters. Both of us bored other people silly talking about our favorite things.

We also shared a rigid thinking style. Sean describes how he built an airplane from Tinker Toys and became enraged when one small, inconsequential part had been left out. Instead of taking pride in his accomplishment and realizing how minor the little part was, he smashed the airplane to pieces. In his mind, you either built the model correctly, or you failed. I had a similar experience when I started designing cattle corrals. One of my early clients was not completely satisfied with my work. I did not realize it is impossible to please everybody. In my mind, his dissatisfaction meant I might have to give up cattle corral design forever. Fortunately, my good friend Jim Uhl, the contractor who built the corrals, talked me into continuing my design work.

Emotionally, Sean and I are very different. I solve social problems with logic and "instant replays" of the mistakes I made, using my strongly visual imagination. I analyze these photo-realistic replays of social missteps as a football coach would analyze his team's maneuvers. My satisfaction in life comes through interests I can share with other people and a challenging career. Sean is a word thinker; he has to figure things out in words and emotions. He feels connected to people via his emotions. Where I replaced emotional complexity with intellectual complexity, Sean strove to gain social-emotional relatedness.

My emotions are all in the present. I can be angry, but I get over it quickly. When I replay scenes, the emotions are no longer attached to them. Sean had a lingering, seething anger I do not have. More like so-called "normal" people, he can get angry and it can simmer like a pot on a stove. In our book, Sean describes becoming jealous of his dog's social skills. It made him jealous that his parents and sister responded more positively to the dog than to him. It would have never crossed my mind to be jealous of a dog's social skills.

However, Sean picked up more social cues than I did. If people tolerated me and did not tease or yell, I was satisfied. When I first started visiting feedlots, the cowboys thought I was totally weird. As long as they allowed me to help work cattle, I was happy. Their impressions of me didn't cause me hardship or sad feelings. To fit in within my work environment, I had to prove my worth by being really good at what I did. I sold my skills and work, not my personality. With Sean, the feeling of "being connected" was more important.

Unwritten Rules contains many examples of the social emotional similarities and differences between Sean and me. However, the basic difference in how Sean and I perceive the world is this: I am what I do and Sean's sense of being is what he feels. In the future, brain scans will be able to identify the differences between individuals' social-emotional functioning. I speculate that Sean, and individuals on the spectrum like him, have a few more social-emotional neural connections in their brain than do I, or individuals like me, with stronger visual, logical processing styles.

(*Unwritten Rules of Social Relationships: Decoding Social Mysteries Through the Unique Perspectives of Autism* by Temple Grandin, Sean Barron and Veronica Zysk won a prestigious Silver Award in *ForeWord Magazine*'s 2005 Book of the Year competition.)

European studies are showing that mindfulness training is helpful for both anxiety and depression. Many books and local classes are available. One study was done by Esther deBruin in the Netherlands. Willem Kuyken at Oxford University, along with other physicians, conducted a successful randomized trial using mindfulness training for depression.

In the old days, the diagnosis was gifted, not disabled. Attitudes strongly influence how we perceive spectrum kids today.

Healthy Self-Esteem

O ne of the most pivotal reasons I think I was able to succeed in the neurotypical world as an adult was because Mother fostered a strong, healthy sense of self-worth in me as a young child. It wasn't one particular thing she did that other parents didn't do. Actually, in the '50s and '60s, consciously building your child's self-esteem wasn't part of the psychology of parenting. Back then kids just naturally did more things together, especially outdoor activities, because there weren't video games, DVDs, and computers to capture solitary attention indoors as there is today.

Even so, I think Mother unconsciously realized two important things about self-esteem:

- Self-esteem is built little by little, through real achievements. For instance, when I created beautiful embroidery, that project took time, effort, and patience to complete and made me feel good about myself.
- The literal, concrete mind of the autistic child requires that self-esteem be built through tangible accomplishments, coupled with verbal praise.

The "fix it" mentality that seems more prevalent today wasn't part of my younger years, either. While I did have speech therapy in elementary school, and would visit a psychiatrist once a month, both of these activities were conducted in a manner that to me didn't feel like something was wrong with me that needed "fixing." Nowadays, kids are being whisked off to one evaluation after another and go from therapy program to therapy program, some five or more days a week. What message is that sending the child other than that parts of him are somehow unacceptable, or that his autism is bad? I think the intellectually gifted child suffers the most. Asperger's children with IQs of 140+ are being held back by too much "handicapped" psychology. I have told several parents of brilliant AS children that in the old days, the diagnosis was *gifted*, not disabled. Attitudes strongly influence how we perceive spectrum kids today.

Throughout elementary school, I felt pretty good about myself. I flourished with the many projects I created, the praise they received from family and teachers, the friendships I shared, and the new experiences I mastered. When I won a trophy at winter carnival, that made me happy. When Mother had me sing at an adult concert when I was in sixth-grade, I felt good about that. Even during the difficult high school years, my special interests kept me moving forward. I could revert to my hobbies when things got tough socially. They helped me get through those years.

Today, kids are being reinforced for the littlest things. It's setting up a cycle of needing approval for every little thing they do. *The Wall Street Journal* has run many articles lately about young kids entering the workforce who need constant praise from their manager or they can't get their job done. Parents and teachers need to take a look at how they're reinforcing children. As a child ages, the amount of praise he or she receives from others falls off dramatically. A child who constantly receives praise for making efforts into the social arena is going to face a rude awakening later in life, which can negatively affect his motivation to stay socially involved.

It's a Catch-22, and one that needs more attention than it's currently being given.

I wasn't praised all the time by Mother or my teachers; far from it. Neither were other kids. We were praised when we did something significant, so the praise was really meaningful and was a strong motivator. The everyday things, such as behaving at dinner, in church, or when we visited Aunt Bella, were not praised. It was just expected that I would behave. But when I made a beautiful clay horse in third-grade, Mother really praised that.

Parents can start kids on the road to healthy self-esteem by offering praise associated with something concrete they can see or touch or smell. This has real meaning to the literal, concrete thinking mind of the ASD child. Especially when kids are young, encouraging them to engage in activities with visible, tangible outcomes helps them learn the direct connection between their actions and their abilities, their sense of mastery and control over their world. You can't build things or paint pictures or create anything concrete without making choices, learning sequencing skills, seeing how parts relate to a whole, learning concepts and categories. This, in turn, lays the groundwork for more advanced skills to form, skills indigenous to the less-concrete world of social interactions.

Try building self-esteem in your child from the outside in, starting with tangible projects, and your child will find his own self-esteem blossoming from the inside out.

For me, social thinking skills largely developed over time and through repeated experiences.

Four Cornerstones of Social Awareness

A chieving social success is dependent upon certain core attributes of the person with ASD. In our book, *Unwritten Rules of Social Relationships*, my co-author Sean Barron and I introduce four aspects of thinking and functioning we think contribute the most to successful social awareness and social interactions. These Four Cornerstones of Social Awareness are:

- *Perspective-taking:* the ability to put ourselves in another person's shoes—to understand that people can have similar or different viewpoints, emotions, and responses from our own. At an even more basic level is acknowledging that people exist and that they are sources of information to help us make sense of the world.

- *Flexible thinking:* the ability to accept change and be responsive to changing conditions and the environment; the mental ability to notice and process alternatives in both thought and actions; the ability to compare, contrast, evaluate.

- *Positive self-esteem:* a "can-do" attitude that develops through experiencing prior success and forms the basis for risk-taking in the child or adult. Self-esteem is built upon repeated achievements that start small and are concrete and become less tangible and more complex.

- *Motivation:* a sustained interest in exploring the world and working towards internal and external goals, despite setbacks and delays.

Often, motivation needs to be encouraged in kids with ASD, especially within the social arena. Let the child feel the benefits of motivation first through using the child's favorite topics or special interests, and then slowly broadening out into other activities. If the child loves trains, teach reading, math, and writing with train-centered books, examples, and activities. Play train-themed games to motivate social interaction.

Based on the social understanding Sean and I have achieved in our lives, we emphatically agree that perspective-taking, being able to look beyond oneself and into the mind of another person, is the *single most important aspect of functioning that determines the level of social success* to be achieved by a child or adult with ASD. Through it we learn that what we do affects others—in positive and negative ways. It's the link that allows us to feel connected to others. It gives us the ability to consider our own thoughts in relation to information we process about a social situation, and then develop a response that contributes to, rather than detracts from, the social experience.

In our book, Sean describes how "talk therapy," as he called it, helped him develop better social thinking skills and appreciate the varied perspectives of other people in his life. During his middle and high school years, he and his parents would sit for hours, sometimes until 1:00 or 2:00 a.m., discussing the most basic concepts of how relationships worked. For instance, Sean explains that even in his late teens, he still didn't understand why it wasn't okay to "absorb" people who took a genuine interest in him and showed they cared about him—that is, why it wasn't acceptable to spend all the time he wanted with someone who was much older and had family and other personal obligations. He couldn't understand why they wouldn't make him the centerpiece of their lives, as did his parents.

For me, social thinking skills largely developed over time and through repeated experiences. The more social data I put on my mental hard drive, the better able I was to see the connections between my own thoughts and actions and those of others. For me, these social equations were born from my logical mind: "If I do X, then the majority of people will respond with Y." As I acquired more and more data through direct experience, I formed categories and subcategories and even more refined subcategories in my social thinking. That's why it's so important for parents to engage children in all sorts of different activities and experiences. Without that direct learning—and lots of it—children don't have the information they need to make these social connections in their thinking.

Perspective-taking works hand-in-hand with flexible thinking; it provides opportunities for experiencing success in social interactions, which in turn fosters positive self-esteem. It can also act as a source of internal motivation, especially as children grow into adults and the type and quality of social interaction expands.

Social thinking skills must be directly taught to children and adults with ASD. Parents, teachers, and service providers are slowly starting to realize the importance of incorporating such lessons into the child's overall education plan. Doing so opens doors of social understanding in all areas of life.

Questions about Connecticut Shooter Adam Lanza, Asperger's Syndrome, and SPD

M any people in the special-needs community are concerned about news reports that indicate Adam Lanza, the gunman who killed the children and teachers at the school in Connecticut, had Asperger's syndrome and perhaps Sensory Processing Disorder (SPD). They fear that this information will make the public think that individuals with these disorders are inherently violent.

There is a wide range of people on the autism spectrum. They range from prodigies—the likes of Einstein, Mozart, and Steve Jobs—to individuals who remain nonverbal. Half of the computer programmers in Silicon Valley may have some signs of autism. However, the vast majority of folks on the spectrum are peaceful and nonviolent.

SPD affects an even wider variety of people. Individuals who have SPD and many different diagnoses or labels may have sensory issues such as sound sensitivity, difficulty screening out background noise, or visual sensitivity to fluorescent lights. SPD can occur in conjunction with autism, dyslexia, attention-deficit/hyperactivity disorder, speech delay, and learning problems.

I have read extensive articles about Adam Lanza on the Internet. Here is some of his history that may be pertinent to his violent outburst.

When Adam was attending his local school, he was super shy and would not allow his picture to be put in the yearbook. During his years there he showed no violent tendencies, and he was really good with computers. His life rapidly went downhill after his parents' divorce.

Adam stopped attending school and became a recluse in his mother's basement. He spent all day playing violent video games and did not participate in any activities except for shooting a gun at a local firing range. He had no other interests.

The gun he shot at the range was the same gun he shot in the video games he played. In my opinion, he was probably visiting some really horrible Web sites, because prior to the shootings, he completely destroyed his computer's hard drive so investigators could not determine what he had been doing on his computer or what sites he had been visiting prior to the school shooting.

What should have been done to help Adam before the shooting occurred?

First and most importantly, Adam Lanza's parents should have forced him to get out of the house and find a job. Whether he liked it or not, he should have been working to develop other interests. He was good with computers, and he could have been working at a local computer store. There is a tendency for some people on the spectrum to become recluses. They have to get out into the world. Video-game playing needs to be restricted to 1 hour a day, as it draws people away from reality.

Second, boys need a good male role model. A good male role model would have dragged this kid out of the basement before he descended into his sick world and began shooting people.

Third, people on the spectrum get obsessed with their favorite things. Teachers and parents must direct obsessions toward positive things that can translate into building careers and fulfilling lives.

There are some individuals, like me, who have extreme problems with anxiety and panic attacks. Taking a small dose of an antidepressant worked wonders for me. There is further information on this in my book, *Thinking in Pictures*.

When I was in high school, I had anxiety and tended to be a recluse. Both my mother and teacher did NOT allow this. They made me get out, be with other people, and develop my own interests and talents.

By themselves, autism and the sensory issues that go along with SPD do not make a person violent. Had Adam Lanza been encouraged to develop his talents and interests, socialize with others, and turn his skills into being able to earn an honest living, perhaps he could have made a life for himself that turned out very differently.

This article originally appeared in *Sensory Focus Magazine*, Spring 2013 issue.

References and Additional Reading

Solomon, A. 2014. The reckoning: the father of the Sandy Hook killer searches for answers, *The New Yorker*, March 17, 2014.

Nagourney, A, et.al. 2014. Before brief, deadly spree, trouble since age 8. *New York Times*, June 1, 2014. *http://nytimes/1jl9ndt*

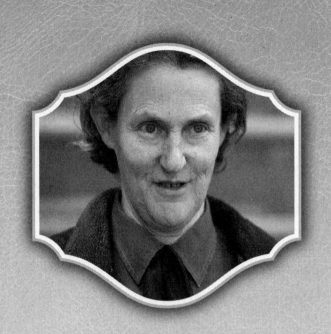

CHAPTER 7

Medications &
Biomedical Issues

Little research exists on long term drug use in children. Doctors and parents need to be doubly careful and consider medications only after other behavioral/educational options have failed to alleviate the symptoms.

I n the early 1900s there were limited therapies available for individuals with autism spectrum disorders. Today, that picture is very different. Autism has captured attention within mainstream medicine (pharmaceutical companies) and within the realm of complementary and alternative medicine. One might assume this is good news, and to a degree, it is. As we learn more about the spectrum of autism and the individuals within it, valid, effective treatment options have been developed. However, not all companies have the best interests of individuals with ASD and their families at the heart of their business. Profit motives run deep, and snake-oil salesmen never go away. New interventions with slick public relations and marketing campaigns attached to them lure susceptible parents with promises of overnight success and, in some cases, a cure for autism. While some interventions are touted as based on research, closer inspection may reveal that "research" was done on a handful of individuals, sometimes carefully selected so that the intended results are achieved. Not all research is good research. Now more than ever, parents and caregivers need to be educated consumers of autism treatments and carefully evaluate all treatment options, especially those that sound too good to be true.

The five articles in this section will help guide you in making good medication and biomedical decisions. You must think logically about the use of both conventional medications and alternative biomedical treatments such as special diets. In 2006, I completely updated the medical section in my popular book, *Thinking in Pictures*. Rather than repeat information here, I'd like to relate some of my personal experiences with medication and biomedical interventions, along with an update on new research since 2006.

In this fifth revision of this section, there will be no great new medication discoveries. Most of the new drugs are slight modifications of old generic drugs. They have no advantages and are much more expensive.

I am one of the many people in the autism community who was saved by antidepressant medication. Throughout my twenties, problems with constant anxiety and panic attacks got worse and worse. I would wake up in the middle of the night with my heart pounding. Going to a new place sometimes brought on waves of panic and I would almost choke when eating. If I had not started antidepressant medication in my early thirties, I would have been incapacitated by constant anxiety, and stress-related health problems. My professional life—the part of my world that brings me so much happiness—would have suffered tremendously.

After consultation and discussion about medication options with my doctor, I started taking Tofranil (imipramine) in 1980. Within a week, the anxiety and panic was 90% gone. No drug can provide 100% control of symptoms and I avoided the temptation to take more of the drug every time I had a minor anxiety episode. Three years later, I switched to Norpramin (desipramine) and it has worked consistently well at the same low dose for over 30 years. Another benefit was that my stress-related health problems stopped. Colitis attacks and pounding headaches ceased. Today, one of the second-generation SSRI (Selective Serotonin Reuptake Inhibitor) antidepressants such as Prozac (fluoxetine), Zoloft (sertraline), or Lexapro (Escitalopram) would be a better choice. (The use of the newer types of antidepressants is discussed in one of the articles in this section.) Since my old drug still works, I am not going to risk switching it.

To keep my medication working, I also turned my attention to supplemental therapies that improve physical functioning. I started incorporating lots of exercise into my daily regime. I do 100 sit-ups every night.

Numerous scientific studies clearly show the benefits of exercise on the brain. Physical exercise can also help reduce anxiety, a common problem among sprectrum children and adults. Living in Colorado, and traveling as extensively as I do, light therapy during the winter months is also helpful. I purchased a travel-sized full spectrum light from *www.Litebook. com.* It really helps prevent the dark winter "blues." During the months of November, December, January, and February, I get up at 6:00 in the morning, while it's still dark, and use the light therapy for at least thirty minutes. This extends my photoperiod to be more like summer, which in turn has increased my energy during winter. I feel so much better.

If I have trouble sleeping, one or two magnesium pills calms me down. It is not a megadose. Each 250-mg pill provides 67% of the daily requirement.

Can I ever stop taking my medication? Countless people cause tremendous problems for themselves when they relapse after quitting an effective medication that had controlled their condition. Sometimes a previously effective medication fails to work when it is restarted. The person can end up in a worse position than before the medication was started. At present, there is a lack of research on long-term management of depression, bipolar disorder, and many other conditions. Funding from pharmaceutical companies mainly pays for short-term studies on medication usage. There is no research to tell me if I can safely stop taking desipramine now that I am 72. Since my condition is stable, I do not want to take the risk of experimenting when there is no research to guide me. I am on a single drug and it works. I plan to keep taking it.

I want to emphasize that the autism spectrum is very variable. Some people with high-functioning autism and Asperger's never experience severe enough anxiety, panic, or depression to warrant medication. Their physical nature, their body chemistry, is such that they can remain calm and level functioning. There are others who need some medication to get through puberty and then they can stop taking it. People with minor depression can often wean themselves off medication, especially if they are getting counseling or cognitive therapy in tandem with their drug use. But people with severe depression, constant panic attacks, bipolar disorder, and people like me—whose body chemistry is out of kilter—are likely to experience major setbacks if they suddenly stop taking medication.

Avoid Medication Problems

A frequent mistake often made with medication use is increasing the dose or adding new medications every time the individual has an aggressive or anxious episode. I repeat an earlier bit of advice: the use of medications is serious business and individuals—doctors and patients—should approach this in a logical, methodical manner. If a drug is no longer being effective, upping the dose is not always the answer. Likewise, every new symptom does not warrant a different medication. A person who is on eight different drugs should probably be weaned off many of them. If they have been on the drugs for many years, one drug at a time should be reduced over a period of months.

Compounding the issue further is that many similar drugs are now available. For example, Prozac (fluoxetine) and Lexapro (escitalopram) are both SSRI second-generation antidepressants. There are various separate yet similar medications in this broad class of drugs. The upside to this is if you do not like one drug, others that address the same symptoms are there to try. The biggest mistake doctors make with antidepressants and the atypical drugs such as Risperdal (risperidone), Abilify (aripiprazole), and Seroquel (quetiapine) is giving too high a dose. Over fifty parents have told me their child did really well on a small dose of a drug but became agitated and could not sleep on a higher dose. For many people on the autism spectrum, the most effective dose of antidepressants and atypical medications is much lower than the recommended dose on the label.

A good doctor is careful in prescribing medications, changing dosage, or adding new medications to the mix. Parents need to be equally educated in understanding possible side effects, changes in behavior that signal problems, proper administration of the drug, etc. This is especially true when medications are being used with children. Most medication trials are done on adults, and while the symptoms in children may mirror those in adults, their body systems are different. Little research exists on drug use in children.

Doctors and parents need to be doubly careful and consider medications only after other behavioral/educational options have failed to alleviate the symptoms. When medication is warranted, sometimes an odd combination of drugs works. (Find more information in *Thinking in Pictures* and the other chapters in this section.) A good rule of thumb is that for most individuals, three or fewer drugs will usually work. This applies only to medication used to treat behavioral issues, such as anxiety, depression, or severe panic, and not to medications needed for epilepsy or other physical/biomedical conditions.

Supplement and Drug Interactions

Many parents assume that vitamins, herbs, supplements, and alternative treatments taken orally are safe because they are not "drugs." This is not true, and caution should be used with these formulations as well. Vitamins are either water-soluble or fatsoluble. Water-soluble vitamins are not stored in the body. The body metabolizes what it needs when taken and excretes the rest through the urine. They need to be replenished on a regular basis. Fat-soluble vitamins, on the other hand, are stored in the liver and fatty tissues in the body, and are eliminated much more slowly. Vitamins A, D, E, and K are fat-soluble. Care should be taken in using these, since they can build up in the system and cause toxic reactions. The body systems of individuals with ASD are often wired differently; their immune systems can be impaired. Parents and doctors should not automatically assume that the recommended dosage on the bottle is appropriate. Trained professionals should be consulted when using any supplement with a child or adult with ASD. Herbs deserve the same cautionary measures, too. While they have been used for hundreds of years, little research has been done on different combinations of herbs or different dosages used for individuals in today's society. Especially when other medications are involved.

The more things used with a child—either conventional or alternative or a combination of both—the more likely a bad interaction will occur at one point. This is the primary reason to try only one medication or supplement at a time, so you can observe its effects before you add another. Some interactions are very dangerous; adjusting doses can compensate for others. One drug may block the metabolism of another. When this occurs, it may cause the same effect as a double dose of the drug because the drug is removed more slowly from the body. This can result in different reactions, ranging from sleepiness to agitation, in different individuals. Even typical food products can affect how the body processes medications, vitamins, or supplements. For instance, grapefruit juice enhances the effects of many drugs in weird ways while orange juice does not. Some supplements act as blood thinners and too high a dose can cause bleeding. St. John's Wort speeds up drug metabolism and it may render vital drugs such as antibiotics ineffective.

I took a soy-based gel cap natural calcium supplement that had strange hormonal effects and made my post-menopausal breasts sore. Now I make sure all my calcium supplements have no soy in them.

Conventional medications can also have serious side effects, among them diabetes or skin rashes. The biggest side effect of the atypical class of drugs is weight gain, and sometimes it is significant. Gaining 100 pounds while on a medication is not an acceptable side effect. For some individuals, weight gain can be controlled by either switching to a different drug or cutting back on high glycemic carbs such as sugared drinks, white bread, and potatoes. Parents need to carefully monitor side effects and drug interactions. Doctors see patients only sporadically; parents see their kids every day. Tell your doctor *everything* you or your child is taking, or any time you add something new into the mix, no matter how "safe" you deem it to be.

Biomedical Treatments

For young children under age eight, I would recommend trying some of the biomedical treatments first, before using conventional medications. Reports from parents and individuals on the spectrum indicate that the single most important biomedical treatment to try is a special diet. They are often most helpful for children who have the regressive form of autism, where they lose language at 18 to 24 months.

Unfortunately, when data from many studies are pooled, the diets fail to show improvements. The problem is that autism is a broad spectrum, with many subgroups. From my own observations, the diets may work really well in about 10% of children who have ASD. They may be most likely to be beneficial in children with digestive and bowel problems.

The special diets seem to work best if started when the regression occurs. However, these diets can be tried with individuals of all ages, not just children. Gastrointestinal problems are often more common in individuals with autism. Pain from acid reflux (heartburn) or other digestive problems may cause behavior problems. Special diets may help ease these gastrointestinal issues.

Special diets can help some children and adults with ASD and have no effect on others. There are two basic types: the gluten-free, casein-free (GFCF) diet (on which you avoid wheat and dairy) and the Specific Carbohydrate Diet (SCD). A special diet is non-invasive, and for some individuals, can bring about remarkable positive changes. However, special diets require time and attention, and in many cases, need to be implemented religiously to truly ascertain whether or not they work for an individual. Usually a trial of one to three months is all that's needed to gauge effectiveness. Some parents notice positive changes after only a few short days on the diet. Others find their child's behavior gets worse for a few days before it turns around and improvements begin. Dedication to "doing the diet" faithfully is needed once one begins. Some parents will try "a little of the diet" and find it doesn't work, when if they had done it completely, the result might have been more positive.

Critics of special diets cite the lack of scientific research to support their use with this population. Literally hundreds and hundreds of parents have reported it works, and a double-blind, placebo-controlled scientific study has been completed. It is impossible to overlook this large (and growing!) body of anecdotal support. Other critics cite the cost of special diets, having to purchase special foods that are often expensive and sometimes difficult to find locally. This doesn't have to be the case, given a little ingenuity on the part of the family. A simple, inexpensive dairy-free and wheat-free diet could consist of rice, potatoes, whole fresh fruit, vegetables, beans, corn tortillas, nuts, eggs, beef, chicken, pork, and fish. The amount of sugar in the diet should be monitored and in most cases, reduced. Olive oil can be used instead of casein-containing butter and all soy products must be avoided.

In general, these special diets are healthy ways of eating. Families with a child on a special diet will find themselves eating a healthier diet, and incorporating more fresh fruits and vegetables into their meals. A new study done in Australia has shown that there was more depression and anxiety when people ate a diet high in sugar and refined wheat, compared to a healthier diet of meat, fish, vegetables, fruit, and whole grains. Some examples of refined wheat products are white bread, snack cakes, waffles, and pasta. If the GFCF diet works, the child must start taking calcium supplements because he is getting no dairy products.

The Specific Carbohydrate Diet differs in that wheat is avoided but dairy in the form of plain, unsweetened yogurt and cheese can often be added back into the eating plan. High glycemic index carbs such as potatoes, rice, fruit juices, and most refined sugar sweets are omitted. This eating plan is similar to an Atkins Diet. The glycemic index for every food can be easily looked up on the internet. Most of the bread substitutes than can be eaten on the GFCF diet should be avoided on the SCD because the glycemic index is too high. Many of these products contain lots of sugar and refined potato starch or refined rice starch.

My Special Diet Experience

Neither the GFCF diet nor the SCD had a positive effect on my anxiety problems. For me, only conventional antidepressants stopped the panic attacks. At 67, my immune function was getting poor and I started getting constant urinary tract infections and yeast infections. I was constantly taking antibiotics and antifungals to control them. Today I am controlling these problems with both diet and acidophilus/bifidobacteria probiotic supplements. Some probiotics contain additional types of cultures and I avoid using them. Dietary strategies have worked well for me to control these problems, and I no longer use antibiotics. Plain Dannon Yogurt helped me with the urinary tract infections and when yeast problems started.

Scientists are learning more about the complex ecosystem of bacteria in the gut. To keep my probiotics working, I rotate to a different brand every few months. This sounds crazy, but I stopped several yeast infections by eating Brie or Camembert cheese. I don't eat this cheese all the time, because I fear that the ecosystem in my gut may adapt to it.

I made up my own simple version of the SCD. I greatly restricted bread, potatoes, rice, pasta, and other foods with a high glycemic index. Drinks or foods full of sugar are totally avoided, since sugar feeds the growth of yeast.

To keep the glycemic index down, I eat animal protein, eggs or fish three times a day and use healthy olive oil on my salads. My diet includes lots of vegetables, salads, whole fruit, and black beans. Animal protein is especially important at breakfast. A breakfast full of low-fat carbs made my yeast infections worse and caused me to get either headaches or lightheaded before lunch. A good meat or egg breakfast with some fat in it along with fresh whole fruit makes me feel so much better. I also never put food in a blender or drink fruit juice. Eating whole fruit is beneficial because digestion is slower, which also reduces the glycemic index. My drinks are water, plain tea with lemon, coffee and tiny amounts of wine. Dairy products are eaten in limited amounts. Restricting wheat helps but I eat small amounts so I do not get so sensitive to wheat that I would have to worry about trace amounts. I have one word of warning. Taking most of the "big white carbs" out of my diet at times makes my stomach hurt. When this happens, I have a little rice with my meat, fruit, and vegetables or eat an apple. The food in my diet is not organic, and everything I need can be easily purchased at the regular grocery store. I have to be really careful about eating or drinking too many high glycemic carbs on an empty stomach. One large glass of juice with 60 grams of carbs caused a huge yeast infection. To get the yeast back under control, I had to eat an ultra low carb diet for a month.

I love sweets and wine. After I got my yeast infection controlled, I found I could have very small amounts of full fat ice cream, wine, or dark chocolate if I always ate it with a full meal. In addition to watching what I eat, I take 500 mg of Vitamin C, a standard multiple vitamin, vitamin B complex, calcium with Vitamin D, and an occasional Omega-3. I buy all my vitamins at the regular drug store with the exception of the B complex, which is Blue Bonnet 100 from Whole Foods. I have to be careful with Omega-3 because it interacts with my antidepressant and I get nose bleeds if I take too much. The Omega-3 (fish oil) supplements have many beneficial effects that are now documented by research studies. Fish oil is more effective than flax as a source of Omega-3. Two research studies show that Omega-3 is useful for children with autism. I get most of my Omega-3s by eating salmon or sardines twice a week. Tuna is avoided due to its high mercury content.

Today I have replaced the yogurt with an acidophilus and Bifidobacteria supplement. This probiotic contains billions of the same organisms that are in yogurt. The liquid ban at airport security made traveling with yogurt in my carry-on bag impossible. I also break open the capsules and dab some of the powder on topically at the site of the yeast infection. Yeast and urinary track infections alternate. Yeast seems to inhibit urinary tract infections. When I feel a urinary infection just starting I stop topical application of the culture and eat some extra sugar along with cranberry supplement. A small amount of sugar seems to boost the yeast just a little bit and it stops the urinary tract infection before it starts. This only works when I feel the first twinges of an infection. If a urinary tract infection becomes established, it must be treated with antibiotics. I also take Solaray Yeast Cleanse, an herbal product for yeast infections. If I have to take antibiotics, I stop taking all herbal (plant based) supplements because they may prevent the antibiotic from working.

Biomedical and Conventional Options

Our knowledge of biomedical treatments and their effect on individuals with ASD is growing. Some biomedical interventions are easy and relatively inexpensive to try. Others are costly and some, like chelation, should be approached with the utmost caution, since improper administration can result in death. Recent research indicates that hyperbaric oxygen is not effective as a treatment. The diets and Omega-3 (fish oil) supplements such as extra B vitamins, DMG (dimethylglycine), or probiotics are noninvasive and worth trying.

The supplement Creatine is showing promise for improving depression. Melatonin is often effective as a sleep aid. There is good evidence-based research to support the use of melatonin for sleep problems associated with autism.

The evidence-based information on Omega-3 is less clear. One meta-analysis showed that Omega-3 was helpful for ADHD. I hypothesize that the lack of evidence for autism may be due to Omega-3 only being helpful when the child's diet is deficient in Omega-3. Studies show that a deficiency of Omega-3 is associated with faulty emotional processing.

There is a need for good research on biomedical treatments, as they work differently in different autism subtypes. Until that comes about, parents should carefully weigh the pros and cons of any biomedical option, and add in new biomedical interventions one at a time, to gauge effectiveness.

The *sensible* use of *both* conventional and alternative biomedical treatment has worked well for me. Each child and family is different, however, and parents should never use biomedical options or conventional medication because "everyone is doing it." I am a really practical person and knew that if I was going to use an alternative method like a special diet, I had to figure out how to do that without it interfering with my work or my extensive travel schedule, and without costing me a fortune. With some research and planning, parents can find ways to test out various options on their child, too.

Tips on Finding Information

It is best to base treatment decisions on well-done scientific studies that have been published in respected, peer-reviewed medical journals. This is what doctors call "evidence-based medicine." Unfortunately, the majority of options available now for treating the challenges associated with autism spectrum disorders have no or limited evidence of this quality to support them. Parents, nonetheless, are trying these options in their search for ways to help their child. When peer-reviewed research has not been done on a particular treatment option, what's a parent to do? Valuable information can be gleaned by talking to parents, teachers, and individuals on the autism spectrum. The tip on eating meat or eggs three times a day came from a friend who had an uncontrollable yeast infection that could not be stopped with conventional medication. I trust information from sources where there is no conflict of interest with somebody trying to sell me something. This principle applies to both conventional and alternative medicine. Because a professional is an M.D. does not eliminate personal bias, nor less-than-ethical behavior. It is common knowledge now that doctors accept all sorts of "incentives"—including monthly bonuses—for prescribing certain drugs over others. Parents *must* become educated consumers and question, investigate, and evaluate any drug or alternative treatment recommended for their child.

Another principle I use in decision making is that the more expensive, invasive, or hazardous a potential treatment is, the more documented proof I need that it is effective. I will try a simple dietary change based on a friend's recommendation, but I am not going to spend thousands of dollars or do something potentially hazardous because a friend said I should try it. Back in 1980 when I started taking Tofranil to control my anxiety, few doctors knew that antidepressants worked for anxiety and panic attacks. I had read about the early research in a popular magazine. My next step was to find scientific journal articles before I asked my doctor to put me on Tofranil. And even then, it was a decision we discussed and both agreed upon.

Today, finding medical information on the internet is easy. Not all of it is reliable. There is lots of rubbish and hucksters selling snake oil mixed in with the really useful information. To avoid this, you can search scientific articles on Pubmed, Google Scholar, or Science Direct. To find these sites, type their names into Google. Pubmed will give you free summaries of journal articles from the National Library of Medicine. Google Scholar searches scientific information and filters out most commercial websites. Science Direct is another scientific search site similar to Google Scholar.

Another great source is Research Gate. It can lead to lots of free articles. Some of the websites where parents and patients chat can also provide useful tips and information.

When I cannot find scientific journal articles, I have a rule for evaluating some of the more exotic, expensive, or hazardous treatments. It is the three family or three individuals rule. I have to find three families who can convince me the treatment works after thirty minutes of detailed questioning. The first question I ask is, "Did you start another therapy such as a diet or ABA at the same time you started the treatment X?" If they say yes, I have no way of knowing that the therapy in question worked. The next part of my questioning seeks specific descriptions of behavior changes. I will not accept vague "it made him better" answers. I want specifics such as "within two weeks he went from ten words to over seventy-five words" or "tantrums went from five a day to one a week." If the family cannot provide these kinds of answers, then it is likely the beneficial effect of the therapy is wishful thinking or perhaps came about because of the placebo effect (improvement resulting from the increased attention given to the child during the treatment period). In doing this informal research of my own, I have found not just three, but numerous families and individuals who have obtained positive effects from using special diets, Irlen lenses, and some supplements. For some of the more exotic treatments, I have not been able to find three families; all I find are salesmen and often extremely costly treatments. It is important to keep an open mind in considering new biomedical options, or in using conventional medications, but in the end, the adage still applies: "Buyer Beware."

Additional Reading

Adams, J.B., Audhya, T., McDonough S., et al. 2011. Effects of vitamins and mineral supplements on children and adults with autism. *BMC Pediatrics* 11:111.

Ammingen, G.P. et al. 2007. Omega-3 fatty acid supplementation in children with autism: A double-blind randomized, placebo-controlled pilot study. *Biological Psychiatry* 61: 551-553.

Bloch, M.H., Qawasm, A. 2011. Omega-3 fatty acids supplementation for the children with attention deficient/hyperactivity disorders symptomatology: systematic review and meta-analysis. *Journal American Academy of Child and Adolescent Psychiatry.* 50: 991-1000.

Bock, K., and C. Stauth. 2007. *Healing the New Childhood Epidemics: Autism, AHA, Asthma, and Allergies.* New York: Ballantine Books.

Doyle, B. 2007. Prescription for success: Considerations in the use of medications to change the behavior of children or adults with ASD. *Autism Asperger's Digest,* July-August 2007: 18-23.

Gow, R.V., Sumich A., Vallea-Tourangaav F, et al. 2013. Omega-3 fatty acids are related to abnormal emotion processing in adolescent boys with attention deficit hyperactivity disorder. *Prostaglandins Leukotrienes and Essential Fatty Acids (PLEFA)* 88: 419-429.

Gow, R.V., Vallea-Tourangaav F., Crawford, M. A., et al. 2013. Omega-3 fatty acids are inversely related to callous unemotinal traits in adolescent boys with ADHD. *Prostaglandins Leukotrienes and Essential Fatty Acids (PLEFA)* 88: 411416.

Grandin, T. 2006. *Thinking in Pictures* (Expanded Edition). New York: Vintage/Random House.

Knivsberg, A.M., K.L. Reichelt, T. Hoien, and M. Nodland. 2002. A randomized, controlled study of dietary intervention in autistic syndromes. *Nutritional Neuroscience* 5: 251-261.

Lindsay, R., and M.G. Aman. 2003. Pharmacologic therapies and treatment for autism. *Pediatric Annals* 32: 671-676.

Lespérance F., Frasure-Smith N., St-André E., et al. 20112010. The efficacy of omega-3 supplementation for major depression: a randomized controlled trial. *Journal of Clinical Psychiatry.* 72: 1054-1062.

Mertz, G., and E. Bazelon. 2007. When less may be more: Searching for the optimal medication dosage. *Autism Asperger's Digest*, NovemberDecember 2007: 52-55.

Pierluigi P., Mateo R., Enzo E. et al. 2013. Randomized placebo controlled trials of Omega-3 polysaturated fatty acids for psychiatric disorder. A review of current literature. *Current Drug Discovery Technologies* 10: 245-25?

Yoon L. I., Kim T. S., Hwang J., et al. 2012. A randomized double blind placebo controlled trials of oral creatine monohydrate augmentation for enhanced response to a selective reuptake inhibitor in women with major depressive disorders. *American Journal of Psychiatry.* 169: 937-945.

Zhang, J., Mayton, M. R., Wheeler, J. J. 2013. Effectiveness of gluten-free and casein-free diets for individuals with autism spectrum disorders: an evidence-based research synthesis. *Education and Training in Autism and Developmental Disabilities.* 48: 276-287.

I like the "à la carte" approach. Use a few items from both sectors of medicine (alternative and conventional) that really work for you; discontinue items that do not.

Alternative Versus Conventional Medicine

Many people make the mistake of taking sides in the debate between conventional medications and alternative treatments, such as special diets or vitamin supplements. Being a practical person, I think the best approach is to pick the item(s) from each that work best for you or your child. One of the most problematic mistakes specialists in the autism field can make is becoming too wedded to their favorite theory. The debate over the benefits of conventional medication versus so-called "natural" or "biomedical" treatments has turned into a hotly contested issue. I advise you to ignore all the rhetoric and logically figure out what works for your child. The way I see it, this is the truly scientific approach to helping your child. Here's a good rule to follow: if a treatment is either very expensive or possibly dangerous, then it should only be utilized if it is supported by rigorous scientific studies.

CBD Oil (Cannabidiol)

There is great interest now in CBD oil. This is a derivative of marijuana or hemp that has the THC removed, preventing it from making you high. It is legal in many (but not all) states in the US, and in several countries globally. Cannabidiol has been found to be effective in treating severe uncontrollable epileptic seizures, and there is increasing evidence that it may be helpful for both autism and ADHD. Some people on the autism spectrum even smoke marijuana to relieve their anxiety. This should be avoided in children and teenagers; there is evidence that the THC in marijuana may be very bad for the developing brain. The brain does not become fully developed until age twenty-five, so until this age, it is recommended to avoid marijuana and products that contain high amounts of THC. It is also never recommended to consume CBD oil, or any other oil-based substance, through a vape pen. This can cause severe, permanent lung damage.

First-Person Reports on Combining Conventional and Alternative Methods

I have observed individuals who responded very well to a combination of conventional medicine and alternative treatments. The most famous case is that of Donna Williams, an individual with autism and author of the books *Nobody Nowhere* and *Somebody Somewhere*. Over the years, I have observed Donna at several conferences. During her early years, she could not tolerate the noise and clapping at a large conference.

When I first talked to Donna, she told me that Irlen lenses and a gluten- and casein-free (GFCF) diet had helped reduce her severe sensory problems. At that time, Donna was an avid believer in the use of alternative methods instead of conventional medications.

At the 2002 World Autism Conference in Australia, Donna told the audience that she had added a tiny dose, just one-quarter of a milligram, of risperidone to her daily regime. The combination of a small dose of medicine along with the special diet really brought about additional positive changes for her. One case report showed that risperidone may reduce sound sensitivity; that may explain why Donna can now tolerate large, noisy places.

I know another person who was helped greatly by a combination of Irlen lenses, the GFCF diet, and sertraline. Sertraline was used initially; the lenses were added a year later. The glasses really helped her organize her writing and do better school work. This was not the placebo effect because initially, she thought that colored glasses were "stupid." Today, she loves them. About a year after the glasses were introduced, she implemented the GFCF diet, resulting in further improvements. Eventually, while she remained strictly gluten-free, she has been able to add dairy products back into her diet. Like Donna, this woman continues to use conventional medicine, diet, and Irlen lenses successfully.

Sensible Approach

There is such a thing as going overboard: taking every supplement in the health food store, for example, would be really foolish. I like the "à la carte" approach. Use a few items from both sectors of medicine that really work for you; discontinue the items that do not. For me, the GFCF diet had no effect on my anxiety, but I prevent a lightheaded, dizzy sensation by eating some animal protein every day. I also take conventional antidepressant medication.

I have found a combination that works well for me. With some experimentation, you can find what works best for you or your child, too. It's worth the effort.

Supplements and Diets

Scientific evidence has started to corroborate that there are specific conditions where natural treatments are effective. Dr. Dienke Bos in the

Netherlands has found that dietary omega-3 fatty acids have improved ADHD symptoms. A review of some of the new research on omega-3 indicated a small, positive effect on hyperactivity. There is also some new evidence that omega-3 oils may help treat major depression in adults, as some cases suggest depression can be linked to low-grade inflammation. Fish oil and other anti-inflammatory drugs, such as aspirin and celecoxib, are sometimes helpful. Many parents have reported that the casein- and gluten-free diet is helpful. In some children, going off the diet caused a really bad reaction. There is a subgroup of individuals who respond really well. One study showed that a modified ketogenic diet with MCT (coconut) oil had some benefits, too. Common problems for many children and adults with autism include difficulty sleeping and gastrointestinal (GI) problems. A randomized trial of a sustained-release melatonin improved sleep, and three new studies showed that probiotics may be helpful in individuals with GI issues.

References and Additional Reading

Appleton, Katherine M, Hannah M Sallis, Rachel Perry, Andrew R Ness, and Rachel Churchill. 2015. "Omega 3 Fatty Acids for Depression in Adults." Cochrane Database of Systematic Reviews. https://doi.org/10.1002/14651858.CD004692.pub4.

Arteaga-Henriquez, G. et al. (2019) Low grade inflammation as a predictor of antidepressant and anti-inflammatory therapy response in MDD (major depressive disorder), Patients: A systematic Review of the Literature, *Frontiers in Psychiatry*, 10:458.

Baur, I. et al., 2014. Does omega-3 fatty acid supplementation enhance neural efficiency? A review of the literature, *Human Psychopharmacology*, 29:8-18.

Banchel, D.A. et al. (2019) Oral cannabidiol (CBD) use in children with autism spectrum disorder to treat co-morbiditics, *Frontiers in Pharmacology*, doi:10.3389/fphar.2018.0151.

Cheng, Y.S. et al. (2017) Supplementation with Omega 3 fatty acids may improve hyper activity, lethargy and stereotypy in children with autism spectrum disorder: A meta-analysis of randomized controlled trials, *Neuropsychiatry Disorders Treatment*, 13:2531-2543.

Cooper, R.E. et al. (2017) Cannabinoids (CBD) in attention-deficit/hyperactivity disorder: A randomized controlled trial, *European Pharmacology*, 27:795-808.

Devinsky, O. et al. (2017) Trial of cannabidiol (CBD) for drug resistant seizures in Dravet syndrome, *New England Journal of Medicine*, 376:2011-2020.

Eaton, W.E. (2015) Improvement in psychotic symptoms after a gluten-free diet in a boy with complex autoimmune illness, *American Journal of Psychiatry*, 172:219-221.

Ghanizadeh, A. (2009) Does risperidone improve hyperacusis in children with autism? *Pharmacology Bulletin* 42:108-110.

Granpeesheh, D. et al. (2010) controlled evaluation of the effects of hyperbaric oxygen therapy on the behavior of 16 children with autism spectrum disorders, *Journal of Autism and Developmental Disorders* Epub).

Infant m' et al. (2018) Omega 3-PUFAs and Vitamin D co-supplementation as a safe-effective therapeutic approach for core symptoms of autism spectrum disorder: Case report and literature review, *Nutritional Neuroscience*, December 13, 2018.

Lee, R.W. et al. (2018) A modified ketogenic gluten free diet with MCT (coconut oil) improves behavior in children with autism spectrum disorder, *Physiology and Behavior*, 188:205-211.

Lui, J. et al. (2019) Probiotic therapy for treating behavioral and gastrointestinal symptoms in autism spectrum disorder: A systematic review of clinical trials, *Current Medical Science*, 39:173-184.

Lui, Y.W. et al. (2019) Effects of lactobacillus plantarum PS128 on children with autism spectrum disorder in Taiwan: A randomized double-blind placebo-controlled trial, *Nutrients* 11(4):820.

Maris, A. et al. (2018) Melatonin for insomnia in patients with autism, *Child Adolescent Psychopharmacology*, 28:699-710.

Mulloy, A. et al. (2010) Gluten free and casein free diets in the treatment of autism spectrum disorder, *Research in Autism Spectrum Disorders*, 4:328-339.

Navarro, F. et al. (2016) Can probiotics benefit children with autism spectrum disorder? *World Journal of Gastroenterology*, 22:10093-10102.

Orr, C. et al. (2019) Gray matter volume differences with extremely low levels of cannabis use in adolescents, *Journal of Neuroscience* doi:10.1523/jneurosci.3375-17.2018.

Polag, S. et al. (2019) Cannibidiol (CBD) as a suggested candidate for treatment of autism spectrum disorder, *Progress in Neuro-Psychopharmacology and Biological Psychiatry*, 89:90-96.

Posar, A. and Viscotti, P. (2018) Omega 3 supplementation in autism spectrum disorder: A still open question, *Journal of Pediatric Neuroscience*, 11:225-227.

Rucklidge, J.J. (2014) Vitamin-mineral treatment of attention deficit hyperactivity disorder in adults: A double blind study randomized placebo controlled trial, *BJ Psych* doi: 10.1192/bjp.bp.113.132.

Sakulchit, T. et al. (2017) Hyperbaric oxygen therapy for children with autism spectrum disorder, CFP-MFC, The official journal of the College of Family Physicians in Canada, 63:446-448 (Not recommended).

Schleider, L.B.L. et al. (2019) Real life experience of medical cannabidiol (CBD) treatment of autism: Analysis of safety and efficiency, *Scientific Reports (Nature)* 200.

Shattock, P. and P. Whiteley (2000) The Sunderland Protocol: A logical sequencing of biomedical intervention for the treatment of autism and related disorders, Autism Research Unit, University of Sunderland, UK.

Zhang, W.F. et al. (2010) Extract of gingko biloba treatment for tardive dyskinesia in schizophrenics: A randomized double blind, placebo-controlled trial, *Journal of Clinical Psychiatry*, (pub).

Autism Medical Update

T he new information on supplements and CBD are on pages 248-251. In this section, I will cover some of the most recent information on other medically related topics. Anxiety is a major problem for many teens and adults with autism. Reports from both parents and counselors indicate that anxiety, and sometimes panic attacks, prevent the individual from engaging in activities. When I was in my twenties, I was terrified of both public speaking and airplanes. To get comfortable with public speaking, I just had to do it. Having really good slides to illustrate my talk was also extremely helpful. To get over the fear of flying, I made aviation interesting. Flying in the cockpit of a large plane carrying cattle switched aircrafts from "scary" to "interesting."

In many of my writings, such as my book *Thinking in Pictures*, I discussed how a low dose of antidepressants saved me from crippling panic attacks. There is an excellent review of medications for anxiety in the Kennedy Krieger Institute (www.iamcommunity.org). In this review, they discuss problems with over activation caused by antidepressants. Unfortunately, they do not discuss the use of lower doses. If you try an antidepressant and it causes agitation or insomnia, the dose must be reduced. I also found a good open-access scientific article on pharmacological therapies for autism by Dr. D.W. Coleman in the *Journal of Child and Adolescent Psychopharmacology* (see reference list). There are some individuals who are taking too many medications. Fifty percent of adults with ASD in the Medicaid program were on six or more drugs. It is likely that they are overmedicated. In a paper by Rini Votira at West Virginia University, there is a good discussion of the serious side effects of atypical drugs such as

Risperidan and Abilify. There is also some exciting new research on treatment resistant depression. There are some cases where subclinical low thyroid hormone levels may be one reason. Parents, teachers, and doctors need to think logically about the use of medications. Way too many drugs are given to young children and they may have unknown effects on the developing brain. When a medication is introduced, it should have an obvious beneficial effect.

Seizure Epileptic Factors and Autism

There are several different reasons why individuals with autism or other developmental problems have meltdowns. The first step is to determine if the problem is behavioral or medical. Below are the major causes of meltdowns:

- **Behavioral** – Child has a tantrum when he/she does not get what they want.
- **Behavioral** – Frustration because of an inability to communicate. Give the child a method to communicate their needs.
- **Behavioral** – An attempt to get out of doing something he/she does not want to do.
- **Medical** – Extreme sensory oversensitivity, meltdowns, or violent behavior in teenagers and adults in response to loud noise or sensory overload. Try a low dose of an atypical anti-psychotic such as Risperidone, which is approved by the FDA for irritability associated with autism. Due to severe side effects, try to avoid use in young children.
- **Medical** – Psycho-motor epilepsy – An antiseizure or epilepsy drug may be effective when a tantrum suddenly occurs when there is no reason for it. The individual may scream or hit without

warning. Suspect psycho-motor epilepsy if a meltdown occurs when the individual is in a quiet place just relaxing. These seizures are extremely difficult to diagnose. A trial of an anti-convulsant drug may work. If it works, it will be obvious. A large survey of medication for autism gave high rankings to lamotrigine (Lamictal) and oxcarbazepine (Trileptal) were good anti-convulsants (epilepsy drugs).

- *Medical* – Hot and Sweaty Rage – There are some children and adults where blood pressure medications may be really helpful. A book titled *Hope for the Violently Aggressive Child* may provide useful recommendations.

Interesting New Findings

A randomized controlled trial showed that melatonin is effective to help individuals with autism with sleep problems. Sometimes parents prefer to use natural supplements because they are concerned about bad side effects with conventional medications. These are real and legitimate concerns. However, there are some situations where a medication may be beneficial to the brain. Long-term use of citalopram (Celexa), a SSRI antidepressant, may help prevent Alzheimer's. This medication is often used to treat anxiety.

Causes of Autism

There is a lot of speculation on the causes of autism. Genetics are a major factor in the cause of autism. There are many different genes that are involved with brain development that contribute to autism. Genomic testing indicates that genes that contribute to autism occur in both humans and animals. A question I often get asked is: has autism increased?

Some of the increase, I think, is due to too much screen time and a lack of the formal social skills training. Most children of my generation received lots of social skills training as a normal parenting practice. If a person has only a slight tendency to be socially aloof, that tendency may increase if their activities become more solitary. Both the environment and genetics are important. Many children today have no grit or persistence because they are not allowed to figure things out by themselves. An interesting experiment with rats showed that they were more persistent and successful in getting food out of a puzzle box if they had to forage for their food instead of just having it given to them. Rats that had to dig in piles of sawdust to get treats were better problem solvers than rats that had them scattered on the floor. Children need to be given more time to explore and figure out things themselves.

Further Reading

Ankenman, R. (2014) *Hope for the Violently Aggressive Child: New Diagnoses and Treatments that Work*, Fugure Horizons, Arlington, Texas.

Bardi, M. et al. (2012) Behavioral training and predisposed coping strategies interact to influence resilience in male Long-Evans rats: Implications for depression, *Stress*, 15(3):306-317.

Bartels, C. et al. (2018) Impact of SSRI therapy on risk of conversion from mild cognitive impairment to Alzheimer's Dementia in individuals with previous depression, *American Journal of Psychiatry*, 175(3):232-241.

Cohen, B.M. et al. (2018) Antidepressant resistant depression in patients with co-morbid subclinical hypothyroidism or near normal TSH levels, *American Journal of Psychiatry*, 175(7):598-604.

Coleman, D.M. et al. (2019) Rating of the effectiveness of 26 psychiatric medications and seizure medications for Autism Spectrum Disorder: Results of National Survey, *Journal of Child and Adolescent Psychopharmacology*, 29(2).

LeCleve, S. et al. (2015) Pharmacological treatments for autism spectrum disorder: A review, P&T 40(6):389-397.

Maras, A. et al. (2018) Melatonin for insomnia in patients with autism, *Child and Adolescent Psychopharmacology* 28(10): 699-710.

Reser, J.E. (2014) Solitary mammals as a model for autism, *Journal of Comparative Psychology*, 128(1):99-113.

Shpigler, H.Y. et al. (2017) Deep evolutionary conservation of autism-related genes, *PNAS* 114(36): 9653-9658.

Sikela, J.M. et al. (2014) Genomic Trade-offs - Are autism and schizophrenia the steep price of the human brain? *Human Genetics* 137(1):1-13.

Vohra, R. et al. (2016) Prescription drug use and polypharmacy among Medicaid-enrolled adults with autism: A retrospective cross-sectional analysis, Drugs Real World Outcomes, *Springer* 3(4):409-425.

VonHoldt, B.W. et al. (2017) Structural variants in genes associated with human Williams-Beuren Syndrome underlie stereotypical hyper sociability in domestic dogs, *Science Advances* 3(7)@1700398.

Before you ask for more powerful psychiatric drugs, you must absolutely, positively rule out a treatable medical problem.

Hidden Medical Problems Can Cause Behavior Problems

D r. Margaret Bauman and Dr. Timothy Buie at Massachussetts General Hospital have worked with many autistic children. They both warn doctors, parents, and teachers that hidden, painful, or distressful medical problems *must* be ruled out *before* child is put on psychiatric medicines such as Risperdal. Some doctors may not even bother to look for problems that would have been diagnosed in a *normal* child. They just assume that all behavior problems are caused by autism. Dr. Buie, a pediatric gastroenterologist, explained that 24% of normal children have distressful GI (gastrointestinal) problems. A study of almost 3000 children with ASD showed that 247 had chronic gastrointestinal issues, such as constipation, bloating, diarrhea, or abdominal pain.

At the Autism 2008 Geneva Center Conference in Toronto, Dr. Buie showed videos of three young nonverbal autistic children with terrible behaviors that were caused by non-obvious stomach distress. On the first video, a little girl refused to sit still to do a task. She was in constant motion and would not settle. She also had weird postures, and strangely, she did not hold her stomach. In a second video, a child was refusing to lie flat and kept flinging and flailing about. In the third video, there was severe self injury and a weird "saluting" posture.

All three children suffered from acid reflux (heartburn), the most common GI problem. Although none of them expressed overt signs of GI distress, such as constipation, vomiting, diarrhea, or touching/rubbing their stomach or chest, their behaviors were a direct result of their severe discomfort. Being nonverbal, their behaviors were their only means of communicating their discomfort. Some of their body movements were, undoubtedly, their attempts to alleviate the pain they felt. All three children greatly improved after they were treated for acid reflux. Acid reflux can be easily treated with over-the-counter medications such as Pepcid (famotidine) or Prevacid (lansoprazole). Not allowing a child to lie down immediately after eating, and raising the head of the bed to keep acid in the stomach and prevent it from burning the esophagus, are other common remedies. If brown stains are seen on the child's pillow, that usually is a sign of acid reflux. Other signs include chewing clothing or other objects, or tapping the chest. Children that had gastrointestinal issues were also more likely to have sensory oversensitivity and anxiety issues.

Other Hidden Medical Problems

Obviously acid reflux is only one of the many physical issues that can cause behavior problems. Other GI problems such as constipation or H pylori can also cause pain. H pylori is the bug that causes stomach ulcers and it can be diagnosed with a simple stool test and treated by your local doctor. I have also talked to teachers and parents who reported that their child's behavior greatly improved after an ear infection or a toothache was treated. A severe yeast infection can also make a child feel terrible, and should be treated.

Dr. Bauman described other useful observations from her clinical practice with hundreds of children with autism. She has observed that girls' behaviors are often more likely to get worse at puberty than boys'. I can really relate to this. When puberty started, my anxiety and panic attacks exploded. Dr. Bauman has found that some girls with autism have an imbalance between the hormones of estrogen and progesterone. Treating the hormone imbalance improved behavior. This problem can be diagnosed and treated by either a very good gynecologist or an endocrinologist.

It is heartbreaking to have a child who is toilet trained lose his toilet training. If that occurs, the first step is to rule out a urinary tract infection that can be easily diagnosed with a urine sample. Other possible causes could be GI problems such as diarrhea or parasites. Dr. Bauman has found that some pre-teen children lose bladder control due to a spastic bladder and that sometimes the drug Ditropan is helpful.

In conclusion, it is vital to remember that, with most children with autism, and especially with those who are nonverbal or have limited verbal skills, behavior is communication. Sudden or unexplained acting out behaviors that continue for days or weeks are often the result of hidden physical issues affecting the child. Before you ask for more and more powerful psychiatric drugs, you must absolutely, positively rule out a treatable medical problem.

Additional Reading

Bauman, M. L. 2010. Medical comorbidities in autism: Challenges to diagnosis and treatment. *Neurotherapeutics* 7: 320-327.

Buie, T. et al. 2010. Evaluation, diagnosis, and treatment of gastrointestinal disorders in individuals with ASDs: A consensus report. *Pediatrics* 125 (Suppl 1) S1-S18.

De Magistris, L. et al. 2010. Alterations of the intestinal barrier in patients with autism spectrum disorders and their firstdegree relatives. *Journal of Pediatric Gastroenterology and Nutrition* 51: 418-424.

Genuis, S. J. and T. P. Bouchard. 2010. Celiac disease presenting in autism. *Journal of Child Neurology* 25: 114-119.

Mazurek M. O., Vasa R. A., Kalb L. G., et al. 2013. Anxiety, sensory over-responsivity, and gastrointestinal problems in children with autism spectrum disorders. *Journal of Abnormal Child Psychology* 41: 165-176.

I have observed that the person actually doing the teaching is often a more important part of the equation than is the method.

Evaluating Treatments

E very individual with autism is different. A medication or an educational program that works for one may not work for another. For example, one child may make really good progress on a highly structured, discrete trial educational program. Another child may go into sensory overload in a rigid discrete trial program and make little progress. That child will require a gentler approach.

Most autism specialists agree that many hours of early educational intervention are needed, but they disagree on whether it should be the Lovaas ABA (Applied Behavior Analysis) or one of the more social-relationship based models, such as the Greenspan (Floortime) or Relationship Development Intervention method. I have observed that the person actually doing the teaching   is often a more important part of the equation than is the method. Good teachers tend to do the same thing, regardless of the theoretical basis of the teaching method. They have a natural instinct about what works and doesn't work for a child, and they adapt whatever method they happen to be using accordingly.

If you notice that a particular teacher does not get along with your child, or doesn't seem to have that "feel" for working with him or her, then try another teacher. The two early educational programs that are evidence based are ABA and the Early Start Denver model. The Denver program uses both ABA Discrete trial teaching relationship-based methods. Younger children will respond best.

Change One Thing at a Time

It is impossible to determine if a new diet, medication, or educational program is working if several new things are started at the same time. Start one thing at a time. Many parents are afraid to do this because they want to do the best for their child, and fear that "time is running out." In most cases, a short thirty-day trial period is all that is needed between different treatments to observe the effects. Another good evaluation method is a blind evaluation, where the person offering the evaluation does not know a new educational program or a new medication is being tried. For instance, if the teacher at school mentions your child's behavior has greatly improved, that would be a good indication that a new treatment you're trying at home is working (you didn't tell the teacher beforehand about it).

With medication, especially, parents must balance risk versus benefit. A good rule of thumb with medication is that there should be a fairly dramatic, obvious improvement to make it worth the risk or the side effects. For example, if a medication reduced rage attacks from ten per week to one per month, that would be a medication that really works. If a medication makes a child slightly less hyper, that may not be enough benefit to make it worth the risk.

Many treatments are now available. Some have been verified by rigorous scientific studies and others have not. Discrete trial educational programs, Denver Early Start and SSRI antidepressant medications, such as Prozac or Zoloft, are backed by scientific studies. Interventions such as Irlen lenses or special diets have less scientific backing. However, there are some individuals who are helped by these treatments. One of the reasons that some scientific studies have failed to show results may be because only a certain subgroup of people on the autism spectrum will respond to some treatments. Further studies, especially those that will illuminate what interventions are most helpful to different subgroups, are needed.

In conclusion, introduce one new intervention at a time, and keep a diary of its effects. Avoid vague terms such as "my child has really improved." Be specific about the observed changes, either positive or negative, and make entries at least once a day. An example of a well worded, useful evaluation would be "my child learned ten new words in one week" or "his tantrums went from five a day to one within four days." Good information will help you make good decisions that will help your child in the long run.

The Problem with Short Drug Trials

Recently there have been continuing problems with the use of very short, unrealistic drug trials for evaluating psychiatric drugs. The severe side effects that can occur with atypical anti-psychotics such as Risperdal (risperidone) or Seroquel (quetiapine) are not going to show up in a six-to-eight-week trial. I am concerned that the FDA approved Risperdal for five-year-olds with autism.

Even though it is approved, it would probably be a bad choice for most five-year-olds because the risk of long-term side effects is too high. In very young children, other safer treatments such as special diets or Omega-3 fish oil supplements should be tried first. There are too many powerful drugs being given out to very young children. However, in older children and adults, there are some cases where Risperdal would be a good choice.

References

Dawson G., Rogers S., Munson J., et al. 2010. Randomized controlled trial of an intervention for toddlers with autism: the Early Start Denver Model. *Pediatrics*. 125:17-23.

Eikeseth S. and Klintwall L. 2014. Educational Interventions for Young Children with Autism Spectrum Disorders *Comprehensive Guide to Autism*. Springer Science, New York.

Goldstien S. and Naglieri J. A. 2013. Early Start Denver Model, *Interventions for Autism Spectrum Disorders*. Springer Science, New York, 59-73.

All medications have risks. When making decisions about medication usage, the benefits should clearly— not marginally—outweigh the risks.

Medication Usage: Risk versus Benefit Decisions

There has been much publicity lately about the hazards associated with certain medications such as antidepressants and pain-relieving drugs for arthritis. It has raised concern among parents whose children already use medications, and has made more ardent skeptics of those who already hesitate to use drugs with their child.

All medications have risks. When making decisions about medication usage, the benefits should clearly—not marginally—outweigh the risks. Common sense dictates that drugs with a higher risk of bad side effects should be used more carefully than drugs with a low risk. A reasonable approach is to try drugs with a lower risk of side effects first.

To approach medication decision-making in a logical manner, it is best to adhere to the following three principles. These principles assume that non-drug approaches have been tried *first* and proved unsuccessful in alleviating the challenge. A child should *not* be given medication as the first course of treatment when presenting behavioral challenges. Exhaust other treatments first.

A review of the literature indicated that children may have more adverse drug effects when compared with adults.

- Try one medication at a time so you can judge its effect. Do not change educational programs or diet at the same time a new drug is tried. Allow a few weeks to a month between starting a medication and changing some other part of the individual's program. Keeping a journal of the child's behaviors, demeanor, and levels of activity can be helpful in spotting possible side effects and/or assessing the degree of improvement, if any.

- An effective medication should have an *obvious beneficial effect*. Giving a child a powerful drug that renders him only slightly less hyper would probably not be worth the risk. A drug that just takes the edge off his hyperactivity, but makes him very lethargic, would be equally bad. I am really concerned about the growing number of powerful drugs being prescribed to young children. In little kids, I recommend trying one of the special diets and Omega-3 (fish oil) supplements first, before giving the child powerful drugs.

- If an individual has been on a medication that is working really well, it is usually not worth the risk to change it for a new medication. Newer is not always better. Pharmaceutical companies promote their new drugs while they still have patents. After a drug goes generic, they no longer promote it. Many of the older generic drugs are very effective and cheap. However, use care when switching brands of generics. Find a brand that works well and stay with it. The way the pills are manufactured may affect how fast they dissolve, which may change the way the drug works. This is especially a problem with slow time-release drugs.

To make good decisions, parents need to know all the risks involved with the major classes of medications. The following section summarizes the uses and risks associated with the six most commonly used medications.

1. ***Antidepressants*** (both SSRIs—selective serotonin reuptake inhibitors such as Prozac—and older tricyclics) when used to treat anxiety should be given at lower doses to people on the spectrum than to the general population. Some individuals with ASD need only one-quarter to one-half the normal starter dose. Giving too high a dose of an antidepressant causes many problems such as insomnia and agitation. The correct low dose can have very positive effects. The reactions to a dose that is too high may be severe, and they will usually start within one week after starting the drug. If the symptoms occur, the drug must be either stopped immediately or given at a much lower dose. Researchers at the University of Kansas Medical Center found that low doses of the old generic amitriptyline were helpful. I know many design professionals who take Prozac and they have done some of their best work while taking it.

   However, I have heard several complaints about memory problems with Paxil (paroxetine). Prozac (fluoxetine), Zoloft (sertraline), or Lexapro (escitalopram)would probably be better choices. In a meta-analysis Prozac came out having the best evidence for use in individuals with autism when compared to other SSRIs. However, if you are taking Paxil and doing well, it would probably be best to keep taking it. There are many new anti-depressants on the market. Usually, they have no advantages compared to older drugs. They will have the disadvantage of being much more expensive.

Antidepressants work really well for anxiety, panic attacks, obsessive compulsive disorder (OCD), social anxiety, and racing thoughts. Most antidepressants have a "black-box" warning of a slightly increased risk of suicidal thinking during the early period of use—the first eight weeks on the drug. Doctors usually prefer to try SSRIs first because they are safer. Tricyclics can cause heart problems in some susceptible individuals. Prozac might be less likely to trigger suicidal thoughts.

2. *Atypicals.* Some examples are Risperdal (risperidone), Seroquel (quetiapine), and Abilify (aripiprazole). The FDA is very specific and states that they are approved for irritability associated with autism. The author speculates that the irritability may have a partial sensory basis. The side effects of these drugs are high. They include weight gain, increased risk for diabetes, and tardive dyskinesia (Parkinson's Shaker). Tardive dyskinesia sometimes causes permanent damage that may continue after the medication is stopped. One study showed 15% of children treated with Abilify got tremors or other neurological problems. Discussions with families indicate that in young children, tardive dyskinesia may occur after one year of treatment. There is no black-box warning on the labels of these drugs, but the long term risks are actually greater than those associated with antidepressants. Gaining 100 pounds can seriously compromise health, impair mobility, and contribute to social ostracism and low self-esteem. The risks continue and tend to get worse the longer the drug is taken. Low doses of atypicals should be used.

These drugs are effective for controlling very severe aggression in older children and adults. Behavioral interventions should be used first before employing atypicals to control aggression. The balance between risk versus benefit favors using the atypicals for individuals with severe symptoms. For those with milder symptoms, the risks are too high.

Similarly, powerful drugs in the atypical class should not be used as sleep aids or for attention problems because they have too many severe side effects.

3. **Stimulants**. Some examples are Ritalin (Methylphenidate) and Adderall (combination of Dextroamphetamine and Amphetamine). These drugs are normally prescribed for children and adults with ADHD. Stimulants usually make children with autism who have had speech delay worse. However, they often improve individuals with mild autism or Asperger's where there is no speech delay. Compared to the atypicals, stimulants have fewer long-term side effects, but they should be avoided in individuals who have either diagnosed or suspected heart problems. The effects of stimulants are immediate and will become obvious after one or two doses. Other types of medicines require several weeks or more to evaluate.

4. **Anti-convulsants**. These drugs were originally developed for treating epilepsy and seizures. They are also very effective for controlling aggression and stabilizing mood. Anti-convulsants are likely to be effective if aggression starts suddenly, almost like flicking a light switch. The rage may appear to come "out of the blue," with little or no provocation. It may be triggered by a tiny seizure activity that is difficult to detect unless a sleeping electroencephalogram is performed with no sedatives. This test is very difficult to do in many children or adults with autism. Therefore, a careful trial of an

anti-convulsant may be a good choice, especially if epileptic-type activity is suspected. Risperdal or one of the other atypicals may work better for aggression that is more directed at certain people. Mark Goodman, a psychopharmacologist in Kansas reports that Lamictal (lamotrigine) is often very effective for aggression in autistic adolescents. This is the stage of development where seizures sometimes occur in autism. Other anti-convulsants that often work well are Topamax (topiramate) and Depakote (divalproex sodium).

The main disadvantage of anti-convulsants is that blood tests have to be done to make sure they are not damaging the liver in susceptible individuals. If a skin rash develops within six months after starting an anti-convulsant, the drug must be stopped immediately. Most problems with rashes occur in the first two to eight weeks. If the person continues to take the drug, the rash can be fatal. Many individuals tolerate anti-convulsants really well, provided they have no liver or rash problems within the first year of taking these drugs. Careful monitoring will prevent dangerous side effects because the person can be taken off the drug before it causes permanent damage.

In one meta-analysis of anti-convulsants, researchers concluded that they did not work for autism. The problem with an autism diagnosis is that it is not precise, like a diagnosis for tuberculosis. However, they may work if the individual also has some epileptic form of activity in the brain, in addition to a diagnosis of autism. Anti-convulsants are approved by the FDA for treating epilepsy and for mood stabilization. I have suggested that many families who have a child with severe aggression consult with a neurologist who is skilled at treating atypical types of epilepsy. Sometimes, this has good results.

5. **Blood Pressure Medications**. This class of drugs was originally developed for treating high blood pressure. They have strong anti-anxiety and calming properties. I know design professionals who had terrible problems with anxiety and drug addiction who completely got their lives turned around by taking a low dose of Prozac along with the beta-blocker Propranolol. Propranolol is an old generic that is being rediscovered. The military is doing research with Propranolol and prazosin as treatment for post traumatic stress disorder. They block the huge fear response that veterans experience during a "flashback" and help stop nightmares. Propranolol may help control rage in nonverbal individuals who are hot and sweaty and often sound like they are out of breath. Dr. Ralph Ankenman has a book titled *Hope for the Violently Aggressive Child*. This book describes the use of both beta- and alpha-blocking blood pressure medicines to control rages. Other blood pressure medications may also be helpful for calming or helping a child get to sleep. Catapres (clonidine) works well as a sleep aid. Blood pressure medications have fewer long-term side effects compared to the atypicals such as Risperdal or Abilify. Since they are blood pressure pills, they could cause fainting if the person's blood pressure gets too low. When any blood pressure medication is first started, individuals should avoid driving until they know how they will react to the medication.

6. **Benzodiazepines**. These medications are used for anxiety, but they have many disadvantages. They have huge abuse potential and getting off the drug may be very difficult to do once started. Some of

the most common ones are Xanax (alprazolam), Valium (diazepam), and Klonopin (clonazepam). Usually an antidepressant such as Prozac (fluoxetine) or Zoloft (sertraline), or a blood pressure medication is better for long-term management of anxiety. Dr. John Ratey at Harvard University usually avoids the benzodiapozines when treating individuals on the autism spectrum.

Old Versus New

Many new atypicals and antidepressants are coming on the market all the time. Some of these have minor advantages compared to older drugs. Many of them are slight chemical modifications of older drugs. Often the older drugs will work just as well and they are available in cheap generics. At the time of the second revision this chapter, there were no totally new types of conventional pharmaceuticals on the market or in the research pipeline awaiting FDA approval. Today there are effective generic drugs available for all classes of conventional pharmaceuticals used in the treatment of individuals with autism.

In terms of real risk, the antidepressants and blood pressure medications are safer for long-term health. However, there are some situations where the benefits of Risperdal far outweigh the risk. It is a very effective drug for controlling rage. If it enables a teenager to attend school, live in a group home, or have enough self-control to learn other cognitive forms of behavior management, it would be worth the risk.

Parents must logically assess the risk-benefit ratio when contemplating any form of medication usage with their child. Discuss the medication thoroughly with the child's doctor. Ask the doctor to provide you with a list of possible side effects of the medication. Do some research of your own on the internet to determine how widely and/or effectively the medication has been used with people with ASD. This is especially true when medication is suggested for use with younger children. Both doctors and parents must avoid increasing drug doses or adding another medication every time there is a crisis. I have talked to parents where their child was taking eight different medications and the child was a sedated zombie.

When medications are used carefully and conservatively, they can help normalize function. When medications are just thrown at problems without using logical thinking, the child can be so drugged that he or she may not be able to function.

Novel Effective Uses for Old Medications

Dr. Alexander Kolevzon at Mount Sinai Hospital in New York uses either Prozac or Zoloft for anxiety, and he has patients where extended release Guanfacine (Tenex, Intuniv) or Atomoxetine (Strattera) have been effective also for anxiety. Both of these drugs are commonly used for ADHD. Guanfacine is a blood pressure medication and Atomoxetine is similar to antidepressants. Guanfacine is marketed as either a blood pressure medication or an ADHD treatment under different names. There are old, safe drugs that are being used for new uses. Dr. Theodore Henderson, another physician who treats autism is using the drug I take Desipramine for anxiety. It worked in 80% of his patients.

Additional Reading

Ankenman, R. 2011. *Hope for the Violently Aggressive Child.* Future Horizons, Arlington, TX

Arnold, L.E. et al. 2010. Moderators, mediators, and other predictors of risperidone response in children with autistic disorder and irritability. *Journal of Child and Adolescent Psychopharmacology* 20: 83-93.

Aull E. 2014. *The Parent's Guide to the Medical World of Autism*, Future Horizons, Inc., Arlington, TX

Beversdorf, D.Q. et al. 2008. Effect of propranolol on verbal problem solving in autism spectrum disorder. *Neurocase* 14: 378-383.

Bhatti, L., Thome, A., Smith, P.O., et al. 2013. A retrospective study of Amitriptyline with autism spectrum disorders. *Journal of Autism and Developmental Disorders* 43: 1017–1027.

Brunssen, W.L., and Waldrop, J. 2009. Review of the evidence for treatment of children with autism with selective serotonin reuptake inhibitors. *Journal of Specialist Pediatric Nursing* 14: 183-191.

Chavez, B., Chavez-Brown, M., Sopko, M.A., and Rey, J.A. 2007. Atypical antipsychotics in children with pervasive developmental disorders. *Pediatric Drugs* 9: 249-166.

Ducrocq, V.G. 2003. Immediate treatment with propranolol decreases post traumatic stress disorder two months after trauma. *Biological Psychiatry* 54: 947-949.

Fung, L.K., Chanal, L., Libove, R.A., et al. 2012. A retrospective review of effectiveness of aripiprazole in the treatment of sensory abnormalities in autism. *Journal of Child and Adolescent Psychopharmacology* 22: 245-248.

Haspel, T. 1995. Beta-blockers and the treatment of aggression. *Harvard Review of Psychiatry* 2: 274-281.

Lohr, D.W., Honaker, J. 2013. Atypical antipsychotics for treatment of disruptive behavior. *Pediatric Annals* 42:72-77.

McDougle, J., Sigler, K.A., Erickson, C.A., and Posey, D.J. 2008. Atypical antipsychotics in children and adolescents with autism and other developmental disorders. *Journal of Clinical Psychiatry* 67, Supplement 4: 15-20.

Mehi-Madona, L. et al. 2010. Micronutrients versus standard medication management in autism: A naturalistic case-control study. *Journal of Child and Adolescent Psychopharmacology* 20: 95-103.

Owen, M.R., Manos, R., Mankoski, R., et al. 2011. Safety and tolerability ofaripiprazole for irritability in pediatric patients with autistic disorder. *Journal of Clinical Psychiatry* 72: 1270-1276.

Parikh, M.S., Kolevzon, A., and Hollander, E. 2008. Psychopharmacology of aggression in children and adults with autism: A critical review of efficacy and tolerability. *Journal of Child and Adolescent Psychopharmacology* 18: 157-178.

Possy, D. J. et al. 2008. Antipsychotics and the treatment of autism. *Journal of Clinical Investigation* 118: 6-14.

Stachnik, J.M. and Nunn-Thompson, C. 2007. Use of atypical antipsychotics in the treatment of autistic disorder. *Annals of Pharmacotherapy* 41: 626-634.

When I go out to dinner with people older than forty and talk about tinnitus, I've discovered that many people have it, and it is undiagnosed. They have either tinnitus or dizzy spells.

My Treatment for Ringing in the Ears

I n my late fifties, I got Ménière's disease. This is an autoimmune disorder that can cause tinnitus (ringing in the ears), deafness, and dizziness. It was really scary because I was rapidly going deaf in one ear and the ringing sound was driving me crazy. Fortunately, I never had any problems with becoming dizzy. My first symptoms were ringing in the ears and within months, I had lost so much hearing in one ear that I could no longer use the phone. I was terrified that my other ear would go deaf. The first specialist I went to sold lots of hearing aids and he was going to let me go deaf. A different doctor got the acute phase stopped with the steroid drug, Prednisone. Fortunately, some of my hearing in the one affected ear returned.

The ringing in my ears was so bad I could not sleep. It sounded like constant cicadas and a continuous low-pitched foghorn. Searching the internet I found some clues for training my brain to ignore the tinnitus, which came from the cochlea (inner ear) that had been damaged by the autoimmune attack.

(An autoimmune disorder is a condition that occurs when the immune system mistakenly attacks and destroys healthy body tissue.) One website said nature sounds help so I went to Barnes and Noble and purchased every new-age CD they had. I tried playing many different CDs at night to mask the dreadful din in my ear yet I still had trouble sleeping. I got an important clue from another website that said, "Use of music and other sounds for relieving tinnitus is 'habituation' and not 'masking.'" So I started playing the CDs at night very softly so I had to strain to hear them. This technique resulted in them working better because I had to concentrate on hearing them. I found one CD that really worked. When I put this CD on very softly, I could tune the tinnitus out.

The Brain Cannot Listen to Three Things at Once

I had to figure out why this CD worked. It was a CD that had a combination of babbling brooks with music and intermittent birds chirping. It was the combination of the intermittent high pitched sounds, along with the continuous lower pitched water sounds that made it effective. This worked because my brain cannot pay attention to three things at once. The three things were the tinnitus, birds chirping, and wave sounds. Other combinations of sounds that worked were a wave machine and a classical music CD played at the same time, and a wave machine and different types of music on the radio. I trained myself to use a variety of music and found that non-vocal music was best. I have also successfully used classic rock, and Spanish music, which has words I do not understand. The only music that absolutely did not work was jazz or rap that had a pounding steady beat. In hotel rooms, I also successfully used music on the radio plus the TV tuned to either the weather channel or movie previews. It had to be something that was totally not interesting. Today, my Ménière's is in remission so I can now sleep with no added sounds.

Ménière's Is Common

When I go out to dinner with people older than forty and talk about tinnitus, I am discovering that many people have it and it is undiagnosed. They have either tinnitus or dizzy spells. Several of my friends started a low-salt diet and their tinnitus was reduced. That is all they had to do, and it works for many other people, too. I had to take a heavy dose of Prednisone for a week and then carefully wean off steroids over a six-month period. Today my maintenance therapy is a low-salt diet and a low dose of a diuretic water pill called Triamterene. If I eat too much salt or forget to take my water pill, I feel a pressure inside my ear and the tinnitus will be worse. I also had to stop taking estrogen for hot flashes because female hormones make autoimmune problems worse. When I got my ear problems, I had low amounts of B vitamins in my diet due to being gluten-free. Today I take a B-complex supplement.

Autism and autoimmune problems are related. Many of the people with undiagnosed Ménière's I've discovered were also parents of children with autism. In many cases, the people had been to their primary doctor and he did not know what was wrong with them. When I discussed Ménière's with one lady, she said, "That explains why I got dizzy after eating a bag of salty potato chips." Anyone who experiences these symptoms— tinnitus, dizziness, and increasing deafness—should consult a qualified doctor to discuss Ménière's. If the condition is diagnosed, trying one of the suggestions I've mentioned above may help alleviate some of the symptoms.

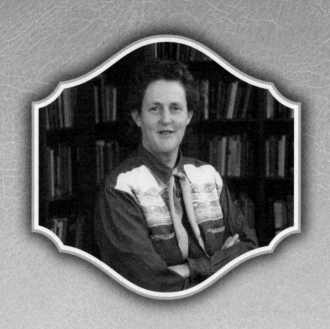

CHAPTER 8

Cognition & Brain Research

I picture the frontal cortex as the CEO of a big corporate office tower. Every office in the building is connected to him.

C ognition is one of my favorite subjects. I'm fascinated by how my thought processes are different when compared to other people's. I love working my mind to figure things out and solve problems because I am a pure techie nerd. Some people share my fascination, while others are fascinated by the emotional/social parts of thinking and functioning. There are four research centers in the U.S. that have done some of the most important work on how autistic brains differ from normal ones: Dr. Eric Courchesne's group in San Diego; Dr. Nancy Minshew,

Dr. Walter Schieder, and their colleagues at the University of Pittsburgh; Dr. Manuel Casanova at the University of Louisville; and the University of Utah group. In my recent book, *The Autistic Brain: Helping Different Kinds of Minds to Succeed*, I cover the latest cognition and brain research. In this section, I will not attempt to duplicate that information. Instead, I want the reader to learn that autism in its milder forms is part of normal human variation.

There is no black-and-white dividing line between a normal brain and the brains of people on the milder end of the autism spectrum. All brains are comprised of grey matter, analogous to integrated circuits that process information, and white matter that connects the processor units together.

Half the brain by weight is composed of white matter "computer cables" that connect different regions of the brain together. In the normal human brain, every region of the brain has cables that converge on the frontal cortex. This allows seamless merging of emotions with information stored in different regions. Dr. Minshew explains that in autism, the "cables" that connect feelings to information may be either absent or underdeveloped.

Visualization of Brain Organization

For me to conceptualize how the brain works, I have to use photo-realistic images. Unless I have a photo-realistic picture, it is impossible for me to think. After reading copious numbers of brilliant research papers, I have summarized them by making a pictorial image about brain function. I picture the frontal cortex as the CEO of a big corporate office tower. Every office in the building is connected to him. Brains are highly variable. They can range from one with a highly connected CEO who oversees everything that goes on in the building, to a CEO with weak connections who lets the different departments do what they want. To put it in computer network terms, the brain is a massively interconnected system.

Researchers refer to disorders in the frontal cortex as "executive function" problems, impairing an individual's ability to process and organize information, create plans and sequences and be flexible in their execution, to self-regulate responses, and achieve goals. Two major factors determine how the brain network will function. They are the long-distance white matter "cables" that interconnect the different brain departments, and smaller local cables that interconnect within a department or between nearby departments. Both Nancy Minshew and Eric Courchesne have done numerous brain scan studies that support this model. In autism, there are fewer long-distance white matter connections and more local connections. More recent literature in 2014 continues to support this model. The different brain departments are less interconnected than in a normal brain. As autism gets more severe, the long-distance connections between departments become poorer.

Dr. Manuel Casanova's work has shown that the grey matter processor circuits are also affected. The brain's basic processor circuit is called a minicolumn. In people with autism, the minicolumns are smaller. Dr. Casanova did some interesting research that showed that the brains of three deceased scientists also had smaller minicolumns, similar to a brain from a person with autism. A brain with small minicolumns has more processors per square inch, and it will be more efficient at processing detailed information.

Cognitive Versus Social Brain

Small minicolumns are connected to white matter cables that wire up local, "inter-office" communication. Larger minicolumns are connected to big, white matter cables that can connect to far-flung offices on different floors of the building. A brain can be wired to either excel at social interactions with high-speed connections to the emotion centers, the CEO, and the heads of departments, or it can be wired to favor the techies in the math or graphics department. In the brain favoring local connections, there would be massive cables draped over the tops of a small group of cubicles to wire together computers that are stacked to the ceiling. This would provide the techies with the computers they need to create really cool graphics or foster mathematical savant skills.

Thus, one type of brain network is wired to handle high-speed social information but is lacking detail, and the other is wired to concentrate specifically on the details. We need detail-oriented people in this world; otherwise, there would be no electricity, cars, computers, or even some beautiful works of music. Detail-oriented engineers make sure the lights stay on and the bridges do not fall down.

People on the spectrum tend to have uneven skills. The local departments in the office building are not wired up evenly because there is a shortage of good computer cables. One department gets wired really well to create ability in art, and another department just gets a single phone line. I am a pure techie, and having a good career gives my life meaning. I've learned to make the most of the way my brain is hardwired, and I don't feel remorse over missing cables into the social parts of my brain. There are other people on the spectrum who have a few more emotional circuits connected than do I, and they may get frustrated and depressed over their poor ability to relate at a social level. Everyone in life has a different set of strengths and challenges within a unique personality. Using a popular analogy, some people see the glass half empty and are pessimists; others see the glass half full and are optimists. It's no different among people with autism and Asperger's; we still share common personality traits aside from the different ways our brains are wired. Not all the "problems" within autism arise from the autism. Some arise just because of who we are and the personality we each have. Michelle Dawson, a woman with autism, has teamed up with Dr. Laurent Mottron at the University of Montreal to produce research results that clearly show the intelligence of people with autism has been underestimated. Normal children tested with WISC (or Wechsler Intelligence Scale for Children) and Raven's Progressive Matrices will get similar scores on both tests. Autistic children given both tests will get much higher scores on the Raven's, an average of thirty percentile points higher. Raven's tests the ability to see differences and similarities in a series of abstract patterns.

Nonverbal Autism

Both nonverbal and fully verbal individuals with very severe sensory perceptual problems report similar experiences: perception is fragmented, or they may see colors with no clear shapes. Sometimes they report that images break up into pieces like a mosaic. In the visual system, there are separate circuits for color, shape, and motion that must work together to form images. It is likely that in very severe autism, even some of the local circuits are not fully connected. Problems in the white matter circuits that interconnect the thinking and movement parts of the brain may explain why some individuals with autism describe themselves as having a "thinking" self and an "acting" self that can't always coordinate together.

Dr. Nancy Minshew and her colleagues state that in severe autism, there are a huge lack of functional connections between the primary sensory cortex and the association areas. To use my office building analogy, low-level employees are able to receive information from outside the building on phones or computers, but they are either not connected or too poorly connected to relay that information to many different departments. Teachers and caregivers of individuals with very severe autism often report that the person has some areas of real intelligence, even though they are constantly flapping. These brains may be like an entire office building where most of the interdepartmental and outside network connections are not functioning, but off in one corner are a few cubicles of normal employees with one static-filled, unreliable mobile phone line to the outside world.

Over the years, I have observed that people on the more severe end of the spectrum are often more "normal" in their emotional/social processing. This can be seen in the writings of Tito Mukhopadhyay (discussed in Chapter 4, Understanding Nonverbal Autism) and others who can type independently and describe their inner world. To return to the office building analogy, there are a few employees in the more emotional and social parts of the office building—the human service and sales departments—that still have phone lines intact and functioning. However, everything in the techie department is broken.

This idea of interconnectivity problems among the different brain departments explains why the autism spectrum is so variable and why no two individuals are the same in their functioning and understanding. It all depends on where the good computer cables hook up. Dr. Courchesne's work shows that there is an early abnormal overgrowth of white matter in autism. As the severity of autism increases, the white matter overgrowth increases. This may leave fewer good computer cables to form long-distance connections between departments, and those connections are necessary for the office as a whole to function efficiently and collect information from all sources.

Is Autism the Price for a Human Brain?

The genetic mechanisms that cause humans to have a large brain may be the same genes that cause autism and other disorders. Researchers J.M. Sikela at the Colorado School of Medicine and V.B. Searles at the University of California have found that copy number variation in the chromosome locus 1q21 may cause both autism and schizophrenia. Copy numbers of genetic code are like volume controls for different traits. A particular piece of genetic code may be either duplicated many times or have copies deleted. Extra copies may cause autism and a larger head, and too few copies may cause schizophrenia. Just the right amount of copies will create a so-called "normal" human brain.

For years, I have maintained that a person's brain can be either more cognitive (thinking) or more social-emotional. A certain amount of variation in copy number would probably be part of normal human personality variation. Too much variation in copy number (adding too many extra copies or deleting too many copies) may cause an obvious abnormality such as speech delay or hallucinations.

Autism and schizophrenia are brain development opposites. Autism may cause the brain to develop extra processing power in the back of the brain for memory, math, art or music; a brain with schizophrenia may not develop enough connections. This might explain why schizophrenic symptoms develop in late adolescence. At this time, a process called synaptic pruning trims and fine-tunes neural connections. Since the network is skimpy, normal synaptic pruning may cause the network to start failing. When the network loses too many connections, symptoms such as hallucinations and delusion may start.

Human Brain Development is Unstable

The genetic systems that have created the human brain may lack stability. The genetic 1q21.1 locus contains a gene called NOTCH2NL. To create a large human brain, it allows undifferentiated stem cells to greatly multiply. This provides more cells that can turn into brain cells. Dr. I.T. Fidder and his associates state that "NOTCH2NL genes may have contributed to the rapid evolution of the larger human neocortex, accompanied by loss of genomic stability of the 1q21.1 locus and resulting in recurrent neurodevelopmental disorders."

Further Evidence of Autistic Traits are Part of Normal Personality Variation

In the animal kingdom, there are animals that are social and animals that are more solitary. Lions, for example, are more social mammals than tigers, leopards, polar bears, and chipmunks. Dr. Jared Reser at the University of California conducted an extensive literature review and found that solitary mammals share many of the characteristics found in autism. Solitary mammals have less oxytocin (social hormones) than those who live in social groups, causing an increased stress response during social encounters. They also have a reduced reaction to social separation from herd-mates. In other words, they have a greater tolerance for being alone. Autism in its milder forms is simply normal personality variation.

Reading these papers was an eye-opening experience. First of all, they indicate that the genetics of autism are also the genetics of normal brain variation in both human and animal social behavior. Secondly, the genetic mechanisms that cause autism are the same genetic mechanisms that gave humans a greatly expanded brain.

Additional Reading

Casanova, M.E., A.E. Switala, J. Tripp, and M. Fitzgerald. 2007. *Comparative Minicolumnar Morphometry of Three Distinguished Scientists*. Autism National Autistic Society, UK (in press).

Casanova, M.E. et al. 2006. Minicolumnar abnormalities in autism. *Acta Neuropathologica* 112: 187-303.

Davis, J.M. et al. (2019) A third linear association between Olduvai (DUF1220) copy number and severity of the classic symptoms of inherited autism, *American Journal of Psychiatry*, 8.

FIddes, I.T. et al. (2018) Human specific NOTCH2NL genes affect notch signaling and cortical neurogenesis, *Cell* 31:1356-1369.

Pennisi, E. (2018) New copies of old gene drove brain expansion, *Science*, 360:951.

Reser, J.E. (2014) Solitary mammals provide an animal model for autism spectrum disorders, *Journal of Comparative Psychology*, 128(1):99-113.

Sikela, J.M. (2018) Genomic tradeoffs: Are autism and schizophrenia a steep price for the human brain, *Human Genetics*, 137(1):1-13.

Courchesne, E., and K. Pierce. 2005. Brain overgrowth in autism during a critical time in development: Implications for frontal pyramidal neuron and interneuron development and connectivity. *International Journal of Developmental Neuroscience* 23: 153-170.

Davis, J.M. et al. 2019. A third linear association between Olduvai (DUF1220) copy number and severity of the classic symptoms of inherited autism, *American Journal of Psuychiatry*, 8.

Dawson, M., I. Soulieres, M.A. Gernsbacher, and L. Mottron. 2007. The level and nature of autistic intelligences. *Psychological Science* 18: 657-662.

Fiddes, I.T. et al. (2018) Human specific NOTCH2NL genes affect notch signaling and cortical neurogenesis, *Cell* 31:1356-1369.

Hughes, J. 2007. Autism: The first firm finding underconnectivity? *Epilepsy and Behavior* 11(1): 20-24.

Miller, B.L. et al. 1998. Emergence of art talent in frontal temporal dementia. *Neurology* 51: 978-981.

Minshew, N.J. and D.L. Williams. 2007. The new neurology of autism. *Archives of Neurology* 64: 945-950.

Maximo, J.O., et.al. 2014. The implications of brain connectivity in the neuropsychology of autism. *Neuropsychology Review* 24:16-31.

Pennisi, E. 2018. New copies if old gene drove brain expansion, *Science*, 360:951.

Reser, J.E. (2014) Solitary mammals provide an animal model for autism spectrum disorders, *Journal of Comparative Psychology*, 128(1):99-113.

Sikela, J.M. (2018) Genomic tradeoffs: Are autism and schizophrenia a steep price for the human brain, *Human Genetics*, 137(1):1-13.

Silk, T.J. et al. 2006. Visuospatial processing and the function of prefrontal-parietal networks in autism spectrum disorders: A functional MRI study. *American Journal of Psychiatry* 163: 14401443.

Wicker, I. 2005. Autistic brains out of sync. *Science* 308: 18561858.

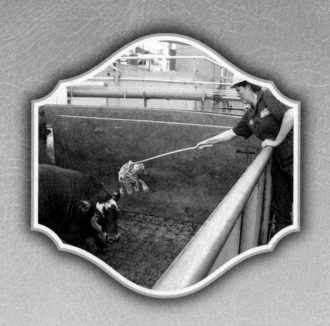

CHAPTER 9

Adult Issues & Employment

*Parents hold primary
responsibility in making sure
their children learn basic skills
that will allow them to function
within society as adults.*

When an individual with ASD graduates from high school or college, getting employment is often a big problem. Many studies have shown that discouragingly low percentages of individuals on the spectrum remain gainfully employed. To solve this problem, work experiences should start before graduation. In the next section, I will describe my many work experiences, which started at age thirteen.

An evidence-based randomized clinical trial by Paul H. Wehman at Virginia Commonwealth University shows that working for a year before graduating greatly increases employability, from 6.25% to 87.5%. To be successful, the program requires a willing and cooperative employer, combined with parents, teachers, and state vocational agencies that all work together. Each student in the study participated in a nine-month intensive internship at a large hospital. The individuals learn to do a job that uses their ability to pay attention to details. Examples of the jobs were setting up surgical instruments for complex procedures or cleaning specialized equipment. Sometimes, more time was required to learn the job, but when the task was mastered, performance was excellent. Students who are slow to learn need to be given an opportunity to develop their skills. The name of the program is Project SEARCH, and the students are now working in jobs at 24% above minimum wage.

There are certain types of jobs that people with autism would be really good at. Laurent Mottron at the University of Montreal explains that people on the spectrum excel at work that involves analyzing large research data sets and paying attention to details. She emphasizes how to capitalize on the unique abilities of people on the autism spectrum.

The way I see it, many of the challenges within this population arise from the less rigid style of child rearing that is prevalent today. During the 1950s, *all* children were taught manners and social rules and "behaving." Mothers made sure their children learned to say "please" and "thank you," knew how to play with other kids, and understood appropriate and inappropriate behavior. There were hard and fast rules to behavior back then, and consequences to acting out were more strictly enforced. Plus, the majority of mothers didn't work outside the home; they had more hours to spend in raising a child and smoothing out problems.

Contrast that with the looser family structures and the watered down emphasis on social niceties that is prevalent in today's society. In many families, both parents work. Proper etiquette is no longer viewed as "essential" education as it once was. Social rules have relaxed and "Miss Manners" has been replaced by a tolerance for individual expression, whether or not that expression is socially appropriate. I don't find many of these changes to be positive, but the scientist within me acknowledges that they are very real forces affecting our population.

These shifting, changing social rules (or lack thereof) make it more difficult for most people with ASD to understand the social climate around them and learn to fit in. Many arrive at adult hood without even basic daily living capabilities—even children on the higher functioning end of the spectrum. They can't make a sandwich, write a check, or use public transportation. Functional life skills have been neglected. Why that is, only each individual family can say for sure. But in general, this lack of attention to teaching basic life skills while children are young and growing, is having increasingly negative repercussions on people with ASD. Quirky friends I had in college, who would be diagnosed with mild ASD today, all got and kept decent jobs because they had been taught basic social skills while they were growing up. They might still be quirky, still considered eccentric or even odd by some, but they could function within society.

One Ph.D. I know is underemployed, but has kept full-time jobs with full health benefits his entire life. In the meat industry where I work, there are older undiagnosed people with mild ASD who have good jobs, with good pay, working as draftsman, engineers, and mechanics. Their early upbringing gave them a foundation of basic skills, so they knew how to act socially, be part of a group, get along with others, etc. Today I see younger individuals with Asperger's who are just as intellectually bright getting fired for being regularly late to work or telling their bosses they won't do something required of their position. When I was little, I was expected to be on time and be ready for school; and I was. Failure to live up to my parents' expectations resulted in a loss of privileges, and my mother was good at making the consequences meaningful enough that it made me behave. As I see it, some of the problems these teenagers and adults exhibit—being constantly defiant and not doing what the boss tells them—goes back to not learning as children that compliance is required in certain situations. They never learned when they were six or eight that sometimes you have to do things that parents want you to do, such as going to church or having good table manners. You may not have liked it, but you still did it.

In light of this shifting sea of social skills and social expectations, how can parents and educators better prepare children to become independent, functioning adults while living in today's society? And what can we do to help the adults with autism or Asperger's who find themselves with adequate technical skills, but are unemployable from a social perspective? We start by recognizing that changes need to be made. We need to be realistic with these individuals and our own roles in shaping their lives. We need to focus on talents, rather than deficiencies.

Parents hold primary responsibility in making sure their children learn basic skills that will allow them to function within society as adults.

This may sound harsh, but there's just no excuse for children growing into adults who can't do even basic things like set a table, wash their clothes, or handle money. We all make choices in our lives, and choosing to make the time for every child with autism spectrum disorder to learn functional skills should be at the top of every parent's priority list. A child's future is at stake—and this should not be a negotiable item. Yet, for some reason, with a growing number of parents, that choice is not being made.

Our public education system also bears responsibility for preparing children to be independent adults. The needs of students with ASD go beyond merely learning academics. They need to be taught to be flexible thinkers, to be social thinkers, to understand group dynamics, and be prepared to transition to adult life—whether or not that includes college or technical school— with functional life skills that neurotypicals learn almost by osmosis. Education of people with ASD goes far beyond book learning. They absolutely require "life learning" also.

Develop Abilities into Employable Skills

Parents, educators, and teachers need to work on using an individual's areas of ability and interest and turning them into skills that other people want and appreciate. When I was eighteen, I talked constantly about cattle chutes. Other people did not want to hear me go on and on about the subject, but there was a very real need for people to design those cattle chutes. The adults in my life turned my obsession into the motivation for me to work hard, get my degree and have a career in the cattle industry.

Teenagers with ASD need to learn how to use their abilities to do work that other people value and need. When I was fifteen I took care of nine horses and built many carpentry projects, such as the gate shown in the HBO movie, *Temple Grandin*. The gate at my Aunt's farm was manual and cumbersome. Without even being asked, I designed and built a gate that could be opened from a car. Teenagers must learn work skills that will help them succeed, such as using their artistic ability or writing or musical abilities to do assigned tasks that produce something of value to another. A teenager with good writing skills could practice these work skills by writing a church bulletin or updating a church website. An individual who is good at art could do graphics for a local business or offer to paint with kids at a local community center or hospital.

In the Education chapter of this book is an article on the three different kinds of cognition. The *visual thinkers*, like me, who think in photo-realistic pictures, are good at jobs such as industrial design, graphics, photography, art, architecture, auto mechanics, and working with animals. I was terrible in algebra and I am noticing more and more visual-thinking students with similar challenges. Many of these kids fail algebra and yet find higher math easy. They need to skip algebra, and go right to geometry and trigonometry. I was never exposed to geometry because I failed algebra.

The music and math minds are *pattern thinkers* who are often good at music, engineering, computer programming, and statistics. Reading is often their weak area. The *verbal word thinkers* who love history are often good at jobs such as legal research, library science, journalism, and any job that requires good record keeping. They tend to be really poor at drawing and visual skills. Most children will usually fit into one of these three categories, but there are a few who may not. Some kids have mixed learning styles, sitting halfway between the categories. One lady I know who falls into the music and math pattern thinking category, understands music from a cognitive standpoint but is too uncoordinated to play an instrument. Many pattern thinkers see visual patterns in the relationship between numbers, but she does it all with sound patterns because she has almost no ability to think in photorealistic pictures the way I do. She has been employed for years doing computer programming.

I also want to emphasize that if a ninth grader is capable of doing university math, he should be encouraged to do it. A person with this advanced level of academic thinking who is forced to do the "baby math" of his peer group will quickly get bored and uncooperative. Focus on the areas of strength and develop them to their fullest expression. A child may be able to keep at grade level in one subject but may need special education in another. Autism is nothing if not variable.

Getting in the Back Door

Over the years, I have observed that some of the most successful people on the spectrum—those who found good jobs and kept their jobs—entered through the back door. They had parents or friends who recognized their talents and learning profile and then capitalized on their strengths by teaching them a marketable skill, such as computer programming or auto mechanics. I got in the back door by showing potential clients pictures and drawings of cattle handling facilities I had designed. I went directly to the people who would appreciate my work. Had I started my job search in the traditional way, with the personnel office, I might never have been employed. Back then my workplace social skills were underdeveloped, my personal hygiene was poor and my temper flared regularly.

People respect true talent and demonstrated ability. A budding architect who brings in a fantastic building model or has a strong portfolio of projects he has completed will attract attention. Employers will become interested in working with people who have ability, even when they exhibit some social skills that are less than on par with their peers. The more specialized the talent, the more willing a potential employer may be to accommodate some differences. However, that is not the case for individuals with only marginal talents. That's why parents and educators need to focus on developing emerging talents to their fullest potential. This provides individuals with the best possible chance of securing a good job in their field, despite their social challenges.

The same principle applies to individuals who are on the lower end of the spectrum. Many successful employment placements are made in local businesses that recognize the benefit of having an individual who will be a dependable, solid employee. People who are nonverbal know the difference between doing useful work that other people really need and appreciate, and stupid "busy work." One therapist could not figure out why her nonverbal client kept having a tantrum when she was teaching him to set the table. He was throwing a fit because he was asked to repeatedly set the table and then unset it, without ever eating. The therapist favored teaching skill acquisition over teaching functionality. A better way to teach table setting is to set the table, eat, and then clean up. All people want to feel their efforts matter, and individuals with ASD are no different. We are learning that a lack of verbal communication does not always equate to impaired mental functioning. Even when it does, individuals can be trained to be contributing members of society. Some of the jobs suited to nonverbal persons are stocking shelves, jobs that involve sorting items, gardening work, landscaping, and some factory assembly jobs.

All individuals on the spectrum, from the brilliant scientist to the person who stocks shelves, find multi-tasking difficult if not impossible. If I had to be a cashier in a busy restaurant, it would have been impossible to make change and talk to customers at the same time. Even today I have difficulty with multitasking and need to work through one thing at a time.

For instance, I can't make breakfast, talk on the phone and do laundry all at the same time.

Parents and teachers, and persons with ASD themselves, need to constantly look for the back door that will open up broader opportunities and employment options. Sometimes these chances can be right in front of you but you do not see them. My first entrance into a big meat plant came about when I met the wife of the plant's insurance agent. That one meeting became the connection I needed to get my foot in the (back) door.

Community colleges have all kinds of wonderful courses for different careers. Many students have found great teachers who served as mentors, both while they were in public school and afterwards. Some parents of talented artists on the spectrum who cannot live independently took entrepreneurial courses so these parents could run a business selling their child's work.

Opportunities are available, with a little creative thought and a willingness to work outside the normal boundaries of education and employment.

Additional Reading

Grandin, T., and Panek, R. 2013. *The Autistic Brain*. New York, NY: Houghton Mifflin Harcourt.

Mottron, L. 2011. Changing perspectives: the power of autism. *Nature*. 479:34-35.

Grandin, T., and K. Duffy. 2004. *Developing Talents*. Shawnee Mission, KS: Autism Asperger Publishing Company.

Simone, R. 2010. *Asperger's on the Job*. Arlington, TX: Future Horizons.

VanBergeijk, E. et al. 2008. Supporting more able students on the autism spectrum: College and beyond. *Journal of Autism and Developmental Disorders* 38: 1359-1370.

Wehman, P.H., et al. 2013. Competitive employment for youth with autism spectrum disorders: early results from a randomized clinical trial. *Journal of Autism and Developmental Disorders* 44: 487-500.

Wehman, P.H, et.al. 2014. Project SEARCH for youth with autism spectrum disorders: increasing competitive employment on transition from high school. In press. *J Positive Behavior Interventions*.

Improving Time Management and Organizational Skills

When I was in college, I did not have the time management problems that are common for some individuals on the spectrum. Since I was motivated to succeed in college, I always got to class promptly and turned in homework on time. In this column I will discuss the ways I was able to succeed in school and life by having good time management and organizational skills.

Being on Time

In my life being on time was emphasized from an early age. When I was a child, meals were served on a set schedule, and I was expected to be back from a friend's house in time for dinner. Every Sunday my family went to church and I had to be dressed in my Sunday best on time. By the time I got to college, being on time for class and getting up in the morning was easy.

A teenager should start learning how to be on time and getting up early before he or she goes to college. This skill could be taught by having the teenager do a job such as walking the nextdoor neighbor's dog at 8:00 in the morning. This would teach the discipline of being up on time for an 8:00 a.m. class. Taking classes at a local community college will be much easier if being on time is learned before enrollment.

Turning in Assignments on Time

I never waited until close to the deadline to study for an exam or turn in a term paper. Each day I set aside time to study and kept up. My term papers were always done way before the deadline. I finished my papers early to ensure a quality job. Doing them early also avoided missing deadlines because of last-minute problems such as getting sick.

Scheduling Time to Work and Study

For me the best types of calendars show one month on a single sheet of paper. I like this type of calendar because I can see the entire month. Monthly calendars are also available in an electronic format. For some individuals a Blackberry or a smartphone has been useful for keeping organized.

On a monthly calendar I recorded times for exams and due dates for term papers. I set aside large blocks of time for collecting research material I would need for a term paper. For writing papers I scheduled time in blocks of 2–4 hours so that I could really concentrate on the assignment. I could get my work done more efficiently and quickly by scheduling fewer big blocks of time compared to scheduling many little blocks. I always scheduled time to study for exams, and I often tutored weak students as a method of studying. I never crammed for exams all night.

Organizational Skills

In the 1960s when I went to college, most students had a large loose-leaf binder for keeping all their class notes. This type of binder solved many organizational problems. I had one of these binders, and I never lost class notes. To keep track of my class notes, I had to have them all in one place. This prevented me from losing them on my messy desk.

At the beginning of each semester, I bought a new binder for my classes. After my four years in college, I had eight binders with the notes for all my courses. Referring back to previous courses was useful and easy to do. It may be old-fashioned, but using a binder is the best way to keep handwritten class notes organized. It is helpful to use a colored tab divider for each class. You can keep a class schedule in the front of the binder.

Today fewer students use this type of loose-leaf binder. If notes are taken on a laptop, I recommend having an icon on the desktop for class notes, and then a separate file folder for each class.

One of the best ways to help a student be successful in college is to work on time management and organizational skills while he or she is still in high school. It is never too early to start teaching these important life skills. If an individual has not been taught these skills, it is never too late to start. People on the spectrum can always keep learning.

Use a Checklist Like an Airline Pilot

I have difficulty remembering a sequence of tasks if they are given to me verbally. I need to make a list of the tasks that I can keep on a piece of paper like a pilot's checklist. The list could also be put on a Smart Phone. For example, the list might include the steps to take apart, clean, and reassemble a coffee or ice cream machine in a restaurant.

Employment Advice: Tips for Getting and Holding a Job

Grooming

When you first meet with a prospective employer, dress neatly. Your hair should be combed and your clothes must be clean.

When I got my first job at a cattle feedlot construction company, I was a slob. Fortunately, my boss recognized my talents and had his secretaries work with me on grooming. Not everyone will be that fortunate; make sure you have good grooming skills.

Sell Your Work

I got my first job because the technical people at the company were impressed with my ability to design cattle handling equipment. Many people with autism and Asperger's do poorly at a job interview with the personnel department. You need to locate the technical people and show them a portfolio of your work. In the 1970s, when I was just getting started with my cattle equipment design business, I always carried with me a portfolio of pictures and drawings.

Today it is easy to have your portfolio always available on a smartphone or tablet computer. I had to carry a large notebook, but today I could have drawings and pictures of completed projects on a phone. Having the portfolio always with you makes it possible to have it available when you meet the right person who can open a door to employment.

I started my freelance design business with one small project at a time. I got additional design projects because my designs worked and people noticed my talent. Starting small and building my business slowly worked for me.

People respect talent. You need to be trained in an employable field, such as computer programming, drafting, or accounting. The technical professions offer more opportunities for employment and are overall well suited to the autism/AS style of thinking. Show a prospective employer a portfolio of computer programs, engineering drawings or a sample of complex accounting projects. It will help. Or go freelance yourself. Many local businesses would like to hire a computer person to come to their business every month to keep their computers running smoothly. Many people who run a home-based business would like this type of help also since they're usually too busy running the business to do these types of tasks. This would be a perfect freelance business for a person with ASD who has strong technical know-how.

Dependability

You need to be punctual and show up for work on time. That also goes for being on time for scheduled meetings during office hours. Employers value dependable employees.

Visual Difficulties at Work

Some people with autism or Asperger's have difficulty tolerating fluorescent lights. They can see the sixty-cycle flicker of the lights and it makes the office environment flash like a disco. A simple way to prevent this is to bring in a 100-150 watt incandescent lamp for your desk. This will greatly reduce the flicker.

If this is not available, try an LED lamp. The use of a flat panel computer display or a laptop is sometimes easier on the eyes than a TV-type monitor. Some people find reading easier if they print text on tan, gray, light blue, or other pastel paper to reduce contrast.

Sound Sensitivity Problems at Work

The noise and commotion of a factory or office is sometimes a problem for people with sound sensitivity. You may want to ask that your desk be located in a quieter part of the office. Headphones or earplugs can help, but you must not wear them all the time. Earplugs worn all the time may make the ears more sensitive, so they must be removed when you get home.

Diplomacy

I learned some hard lessons about being diplomatic when I had my first interactions with people at work. Some senior engineers designed a project that contained some mistakes that were obvious to me. Not knowing any better, I wrote a letter to their boss, citing in great detail the errors in their design, and calling them "stupid." It was not well received. You simply cannot tell other people they are stupid, even if they really are stupid. Just do your job and never criticize your boss or other employees.

Freelance Work

This is often a good way to work because it avoids many of the social problems. When I design equipment, I can go into the plant, get the project done, and then leave before I get involved in complex workplace politics. The internet makes freelancing much easier. If you can find a boss who recognizes both your strengths and social limitations, this will make life on the job much easier.

Being Too Good

Several people with autism or Asperger's have told me that they got into trouble with coworkers at a factory because they were "too good" at assembling "widgets." The problem of employee jealousy is a difficult thing to understand, but it exists in the workplace. The boss likes the hard worker, but the other employees may hate him or her. If coworkers do get jealous of your work, I found that it is helpful to try to find something they have built or done that you can genuinely compliment them on. It helps them feel appreciated and that they, too, have done a good job.

Avoid the Peter Principle

The Peter Principle states that people have a tendency to rise to their level of incompetence. There have been several sad cases where a good draftsman, lab technician, or journalist with autism or AS has been promoted into management, and then fired because the social situations just got too complex. The person with autism or Asperger's is especially vulnerable to being promoted into a job they cannot handle because of the social issues. It may be best to politely tell your boss that you can use your skills best in your present position.

Be Nice and Have Good Manners

People who are polite and cheerful will have an easier time getting along at work. Make sure you always say please and thank you. Good table manners are a must. Greet your fellow workers at least once each day and actively try to engage in some small talk with the people you work with most closely. While it's not necessary to form friendships with everyone you work with, some social interaction is needed if you are to be viewed as part of the group.

Workplace Politics

One of the hardest lessons I had to learn when I entered the workplace is that some people in a company had personal agendas other than doing their best work. For some, it was to climb the corporate ladder and achieve some high level position. For others, it was to do the least amount of work possible without getting fired. Another rule I learned is to avoid discussing controversial subjects at work. Sex, religion, and political affiliations are subjects that should not be discussed at work. You can easily alienate people or give them cause to dislike you when you overstep these boundaries. You may hear other employees talking about these subjects; let them. Keep in mind that the "hidden social rules" in doing so are massive and spectrum individuals usually miss most of them. Safe subjects are pets, sports, electronics, weather, hobbies, and popular TV shows and movies that avoid these sensitive areas. Workplace politics are not easy to understand; just realize that they exist. Try to stay out of it, unless it directly jeopardizes your job or affects your ability to perform your job.

Teens with ASD Must Learn Both Social and Work Skills to Keep Jobs

I have been seeing too many teenagers and young adults in their twenties who have never learned any job-related social skills and the discipline of having to do the work that is assigned to them. This greatly interferes with their ability to get and keep jobs. An individual must not only learn the skills of a trade but also must know how to work with others. Many individuals manage to get a job and then fail to keep it because they have never learned the discipline of teamwork and working hard. Even self-employed people must know how to work with others, or they won't have a job for long. Too many individuals who have much milder symptoms than mine are ending up collecting social security disability payments.

One may wonder where all the undiagnosed older people with mild autism spectrum disorder (ASD), Asperger's Syndrome, or the new DSM-5 diagnosis of social communication disorder are.

I see these people all the time in my work in the livestock industry. They are the old hippie who runs the maintenance shop at a meat plant, the guy who runs the computer department, or a person who is a really good welder. These older undiagnosed people on the milder end of the spectrum have kept their jobs because they learned both work skills and social skills. For some of these older individuals, a paper route was the best thing that ever happened to them. Paper routes taught the discipline of work and the reward of earning money. Today the paper routes are gone, but a 12-year-old could walk dogs for 2 or 3 of the neighbors, fix computers, shop for older people, work at a family business, or be a museum tour guide. Parents need to set up opportunities for learning to work, through neighbors and friends. It is important that the job involves working for other people, outside the home. Volunteer work is also effective, but it needs to be on a regular schedule. Some examples that could be easily set up in the neighborhood are setting up chairs every weekend at the local church, working in a farmer's market, or making snacks for different events in the community.

It's Never Too Early!

Sewing. At age 13, I worked two afternoons a week for a local seamstress who did freelance sewing out of her house. Mother set up this job for me. I hemmed dresses and took apart garments. The main thing I learned from this job was I got rewarded with money because I did the job right.

Working with animals. At age 15, I cleaned horse stalls every day at the boarding school I attended and I took care of the school's horses. I got this job because I took the initiative to just start doing it. Others were more than happy to let me do it. I often get asked, "What motivated you?" I was motivated by the sense of accomplishment and the recognition I received working in the horse barn as a volunteer job. Gradually the job morphed into managing the horse barn. During the summer, mother arranged for me to develop further work skills at my aunt's ranch.

Carpentry and designing signs. At boarding school, at around age 16 or 17, I was encouraged when I expressed an interest in doing carpentry work on our ski tow house. I installed tongueand-groove wood siding with white trim. Other projects I completed were shingling the barn roof and making signs for events such as the winter carnival. From this experience I learned how to make products that other people would like. I had to make a sign that was appropriate for our school's winter carnival. This was a volunteer job and I enjoyed the recognition for making something that other people appreciated.

College internships. I completed two summer internships arranged by my mother and the staff at Franklin Pierce College. One summer I worked with children with ASD. The next summer, I worked in a research lab and I had to rent a house and share it with another person. My roommate and I often cooked together and ate the same things for supper. She loved liver and I ate it even though I did not like it. On another night, we ate something that I liked. This was an extension of the turn taking I had learned from playing board games as a young child.

Magazine writing and design work. During my childhood, I had lots of practice talking to adults. When I was eight, Mother had me dress up in my Sunday best and shake hands and introduce myself to her dinner guests. I also served the snacks during the cocktail hour. I was the greeter and snack server every time Mother had friends over for dinner. When I went to Arizona State University to get my master's degree, I already had the entrepreneurial spirit. I had the confidence to walk up to people and show them my work. The HBO movie, *Temple Grandin*, shows me walking up to the editor of the *Arizona Farmer Rancher* and getting his card. I actually did this. This is how I got my first article in the magazine. This is an alternative to the usual job application process—which has worked for me.

My design business started the same way. It was one small project at a time. When people saw my drawings, they were impressed. It was tons of hard work; it was not easy. But what really helped me was that I had learned how to work and how to get along with others at my previous jobs.

It's Never Too Late!

I want to emphasize that it is never too late to help your child learn these vital skills. Recently, I met a mother whose son was undiagnosed, and the family called him "Sammy who is different." His mother made him get up every morning and get out the door to work. She had to push him. She wondered if she would have pushed him as hard if he had been Asperger Sammy. Today he is in his thirties and has a career he loves.

Teachers and parents need to "stretch" individuals on the milder end of the spectrum. To develop my abilities and social skills, I had to be pushed just outside my comfort zone. One word of caution: the activities that stretched and helped me to develop were never a sudden surprise. Remember that surprises can cause panic and fear for individuals on the spectrum. Be sure to prepare the person for the experiences that will help him achieve long-time job success!

Developing a skill into an employable position will take lots of work and more training for people with autism. However, once they succeed, they will become an excellent employee. But, they must avoid being promoted from a position they can handle well to a management position they cannot handle.

Happy People on the Autism Spectrum Have Satisfying Jobs or Hobbies

I n my travels to many autism meetings, I have observed that the high-functioning people with autism or Asperger's who make the best adjustments in life are the ones who have satisfying jobs. A job that uses a person's intellectual abilities is great for improving self-esteem. Conversely, the most unhappy people on the spectrum I have met are those who did not develop a good employable skill or a hobby they can share with others. With so much of adult life spent in our jobs, it makes sense that people with satisfying jobs will generally be happier with their lives and better able to respond to different situations that may arise.

I have met several successful people on the spectrum who program computers. One Asperger's computer programmer told me she was happy because now she is with "her people." At another meeting, I met a father and son. The father had taught his son computer programming. He started teaching him when he was in the fourth grade and now he works at a computer company. For many people with autism/AS, the way our mind works is well-suited to this profession. Parents and teachers should capitalize on this ability and encourage its development.

Several years ago, I visited autism programs in Japan. I met a large number of high-functioning people on the autism spectrum. Every one of them was employed in a good job. One man translated technical and legal documents. Another person was an occupational therapist and there were several computer programmers. One man who was somewhat less high-functioning works as a baker. What I noticed is that the attitude in Japan is to develop skills. These people with autism/AS benefited from that attitude, and would for the rest of their lives.

While developing an inherent skill into an employable position can be work, it is necessary for people with autism/AS to try hard to do this. However, once they succeed, they must be careful to avoid being promoted from a technical position they can handle well to a management position they cannot handle. I have heard several sad stories of successful people being promoted out of jobs they were good at. These people had jobs such as draftsman, lab technicians, sports writers, and computer programmers. Once they were required to interact socially as part of their management position, their performance suffered.

Hobbies where people have shared interests are also great in building self-esteem. I read about a woman who was unhappy in a dead-end job. Her life turned around when she discovered that there were other people in the world also interested in her hobby. In her spare time, she breeds fancy chickens. Through the internet, she communicates with other chicken breeders.

Because she explored her hobby, she is now much happier, even though she still works at her dead-end job. In my opinion, using the internet for communicating with other hobbyists is much more constructive than griping with other people on the spectrum in a chat room. That doesn't benefit anyone.

Parents and teachers need to place a priority on discovering and then developing the many skills that people with autism or Asperger's possess. These skills can be turned into careers and hobbies that will provide shared interests with other people.

This will bring much happiness into the lives of people on the autism spectrum.

Inside or Outside? The Autism/ Asperger's Culture

A frequent topic of discussion within the autism/Asperger's community is how much people with autism/AS should have to adapt to the world of the "neurotypicals." My view is that you should still be yourself, but you will have to make some changes in your behavior, too. Years ago, Dr. Leo Kanner, the person who first described autism, stated that the people who made the best adaptation to the world realized themselves that they had to make some behavioral changes.

This was true for me, too. In 1974, I was hired by a feedlot construction company. My boss made it very clear to me that I had to improve my grooming. I dressed like a slob and paid very little attention to my grooming habits. With the help of some of the secretaries, I learned to dress better and I worked conscientiously to have better personal hygiene. In the HBO movie my boss slammed a can of deodorant on the table in front of me and said, "You stink." This really happened to me, and at the time I was furious. Today I thank that boss for forcing me to change. It made me more socially accepted. For me, it was a logical process; it followed the *if/ then* sequence of a computer code. *If* I wanted my job, *then* I had to change these behaviors. So I did.

Even today, I do not dress the way everybody else does. I like to wear Western clothes; they are my way of expressing myself. Dressing like this is acceptable; being shabby is not.

I think it is OK to be eccentric. There are many geeky eccentric people who are very successful in many fields. Silicon Valley is full of brilliant people who look and act differently, like the geek Sheldon character in the television series, *The Big Bang Theory*. (If you've never watched this show, do so. The four main characters all have social challenges in various ways, and this series can be used to discuss social problems and solutions with a spectrum individual.) Many people with strong eccentricities are likely to be on the milder end of the autism spectrum. As long as you're good at what you do, being eccentric is often overlooked or accepted by others. This is not the case if the talent level is mediocre or poor. One time I talked to a lady with AS who liked to wear plastic, see-through dresses made in bright DayGlo colors. Her employer really frowned upon this. She told me that wearing these dresses was part of being who she was. While I understood her desire to retain her individuality, I pointed out to her that her dresses might be okay at a party, but they were inappropriate attire for an office environment. Unless she compromised, her job would be in jeopardy. I suggested a toned-down version of her outfits that would be more socially acceptable at work, such as wearing a conventional dress and decorating it with a few DayGlo accessories, such as a belt, purse or earrings.

Techies versus Suits: The Corporate World

In the corporate world, there is constant friction between technical people, such as computer programmers and engineers, and managers. The tech staff often refer to managers as "suits" (but we don't say this to their faces). Many technical people in large industries have mild autism or Asperger's traits. To them, technical things are interesting and social things are boring. Some of the best times in my life have been spent with other engineers and techies discussing how to build meat plants. The technical people are my social world. We share common personality and behavior traits that provide us with common ground for discussion, and help us better understand each other. (It is also great fun to talk about how most "suits" would be incapable of making a paper bag.)

Every big corporation in a technical field has its department of the social misfits who make the place run. Even a bank has some purely technical people who handle accounting, fix ATMs, and run the computers. There is no black-and-white dividing line between computer nerds or geeks or Asperger's or high-functioning autism. And there will always be friction between the techies and the suits. The suits are the highly social people who rise to the top and become managers. However, they would have nothing to sell and no business to run if they lost all their techies.

Parents, teachers, or others who involve themselves with people with autism/AS need to realize that you cannot turn a non-social animal into a social one. Your focus should be teaching people with autism/AS to adapt to the social world around them, while still retaining the essence of who they are, including their autism/AS. Learning social survival skills is important, but I cannot be something I am not. Social skills teaching methods, such as Carol Gray's Social Stories™, are essential for school-aged kids. These skills should be taught early on. But efforts to enlarge the social world of teens and adults with autism/ AS should follow a different path. Rather than focus on their deficiencies, it's better to focus on their abilities, and find creative ways to capitalize on their strengths to bring them more into social situations. Some of the bright, socially awkward teenagers need to be removed from the torture chamber of high school and enrolled in technical classes at a community college. This will enable them to be with their true intellectual peers, in fields such as computer programming, electronics, accounting, graphic arts, and other pursuits. Recently, I looked at the catalogue from a community college and all the different, fascinating technical courses would have been great for me in high school.

Some people with autism/AS think in very rigid patterns, and see a particular behavior in an all-or-nothing manner. When we are asked, or expected, to change a behavior, we think that means we need to extinguish it. Most times, that is not the case. It is more that we need to modify the behavior and understand the times and places when it is acceptable, and the times and places when it is not. For instance, I can still dress like a slob in my own home, when no one else is around (a trait I've learned is shared with many neurotypicals). Finding a way to compromise so that we keep our personal nature, but conform to some of the unspoken rules of society (including the workplace), is where our efforts need to be.

Additional Reading

Silberman, S. 2015. NeuroTribes: *The Legacy of Autism and the Future of Neurodiversity*, Avery Books Penguin Random House, New York, NY.

Portfolios Can Open Job and College Opportunities

I ndividuals with autism spectrum disorder (ASD) need to get creative and find ways to discover employment or educational opportunities without going through the traditional front-door route of interviews or entrance exams. I never sold a single design job in my cattle equipment design business by doing an interview; I sold jobs by showing a portfolio of my work to the managers of packing plants and feedlots. I learned early in my career that if I showed drawings and photos of my work to the right person, I could get a job.

When I was first starting out, everybody thought I was a weird nerd, but I got respect when I showed off my drawings. I got into the Swift & Company meat plant in the early 1970s because I met a lady who liked the shirt I had embroidered by hand. She turned out to be the wife of the plant's insurance agent. I was wearing my portfolio and I did not realize it! You never know where you may meet the person who can open the door for you.

Put Your Portfolio on Your Phone

With today's smartphones, it is really easy for the individual with ASD, parents, and teachers to carry a portfolio. The portfolio can contain pictures of art, drawings, computer programming, samples of creative writing, mathematics, and many other things. In many situations, there is a backdoor but many people fail to see it. One secret is networking with the right person. That person could be a retired engineer, a lady in the choir, or the man in line at the supermarket checkout aisle. This is why your portfolio must always be with you. Countless times I have had young people on the spectrum tell me that they have been turned away at the "front door." I have talked to many talented individuals, but most of them failed to have their portfolio with them, or their portfolio was messy with poor work mixed in with their good work.

Technology Is a Backdoor

The secret is to show either your own work or your child's work to the right person. Today's social networks such as Facebook and LinkedIn make it even easier to find the person who can open the backdoor and circumvent the front-door interview or admissions process. Wikipedia has a list of social networking websites. Use the keywords *social networking websites* to locate appropriate sites.

Access Higher Education

Kristine Barnett, a mother of a young boy with autism, found that her son was going nowhere in a special education classroom. He was bored and exhibited challenging behaviors. She started taking him to a local observatory where he could look through a telescope and listen to fascinating lectures. She bought him advanced books on astronomy, and he learned algebra in elementary school. Kristine recognized the need to keep Jake in a regular elementary school class so he could learn social skills. To prevent boredom, he was allowed to read his higher-level math books when the other children were doing arithmetic. When Jake was eight, Kristine called an astronomy professor at the local university and asked if Jake could sit in on a lecture. Jake impressed the professor with his knowledge, and other professors became interested in him. Jake quickly advanced through college math and physics classes. Jake's story is an excellent example of getting in the backdoor.

Make It Easy for Others to Help

Every week I receive numerous inquiries from people on the spectrum, parents, and teachers who are begging for help. The problem is that many of them make it difficult for me to reach them. I get letters where the only contact information is on the envelope, and I cannot read it. I get emails that do not have phone numbers and postal addresses. You must include complete information if you want to get through to a busy person. You need to make it easy to contact you. Correspondence is often answered on weekends by busy people so give your cell phone number. Due to viruses, many people will not open a strange email attachment, so you need to establish contact via the phone or email first.

After seeing a person's strong portfolio, a top professor in math, art, physics, or creative writing who believes in that student will find a way to get him into the university even though that student may have failed in other academic areas. Individuals have been accepted into good college programs because they showed their portfolio to the right professor.

Resource

Barnett, Kristine. 2013. *The Spark: A Mother's Story of Nurturing Genius.* New York: Random House.

Going to College: Tips for People with Autism & Asperger's

Going off to college can be an unnerving experience for people with autism and Asperger's. Usually the high level of help that parents and teachers provide during middle and high school just drops off, and the person can find the transition difficult at best. In this column, I'll share some tips I learned from my college experience.

Teasing

When I was in high school, being teased was torture. Teenagers were hyper-social beings I did not understand. I think that some autistic or Asperger's students who are capable of doing college level work need to be removed from the difficult high school scene. Let them take a few courses at a community college or university. Parents often ask about age restrictions at the college; I learned a long time ago it is better not to ask. Just sign up the student.

Tutors and Mentors

I had a great science teacher when I was in high school. When the teasing became unbearable, I did science projects in Mr. Carlock's lab. He was often there to help me when I enrolled in college. Having the same mentor in both high school and college was a tremendous help. I have talked to many students who failed several classes and dropped out of school because they did not seek help or tutoring when they started having trouble with a subject. Seek help at the first sign of trouble. When I had difficulty with math and French class, I found people to tutor me. It made the difference between me failing and succeeding.

Uneven Skills

Many people on the autism continuum have uneven skills. They do well in some subjects and poorly in others. Tutoring may be needed in some subjects. It also may be a good idea to take a lighter course load.

Living at College

My first room assignment in college was with two other roommates. This was a disaster. I could not sleep and I had no peace and quiet. I was then moved to a room with one roommate. This was a much better arrangement. Several of the roommates and I became good friends. A person with autism or Asperger's needs a quiet place to live. I recommend visiting the campus before enrolling to make the transition easier.

Campus Clubs

I was active in several campus organizations where I was able to use my skills and talents. People appreciate talent, and being good at something helps compensate for being weird. When the college put on a musical variety show, I made many of the sets. I also made signs and posters for the ski club and the social committee.

Tips on Classes

I always sat in the front row so I could hear better. It is sometimes difficult for me to hear hard consonant sounds. After class, I always recopied all my notes to help me learn the material. Fluorescent lights did not bother me, but many people with autism or Asperger's cannot tolerate them. The room will appear to flash on and off like a disco, which makes learning during a lecture difficult. Some students have found that placing a lamp next to their chair with an old-fashioned incandescent bulb will help reduce the flicker effect. Wearing a baseball cap with a long visor helps make the fluorescent ceiling lights more tolerable. Audio-record the lecture so it can be listened to later in a room without distractions.

Smaller colleges and college classes may be a better choice for some students with ASD. I went to a small college that had small classes. That was a real benefit, as it gave me better access to my instructors and removed the intense sensory problems of a large classroom with hundreds of people. For some students, taking the first two years of classes at a community college may help prevent them from being overwhelmed by college experiences and either dropping out or flunking out.

Behavior in Class

There are certain "expected" behaviors of students while they are in a classroom setting. Often these "unwritten rules" are not taught to a student before college. Two big classroom behavior no-no's are monopolizing the teachers' time and disrupting the class. For instance, I had a rule that I could ask a maximum of two questions per class period. I know of many spectrum students who will monopolize a teacher's time with an endless stream of questions, or who will interrupt others who are speaking in class to challenge what they are saying. These are both inappropriate behaviors. Others include making excessive noise while others are trying to concentrate (like during an exam), talking on a cellphone during class, listening to music on an iPod during class, etc. Spectrum students who are not aware of these hidden rules can ask the instructor or a fellow classmate for some help. Don't assume you know these rules innately.

Grooming Skills

You have to learn to not be a slob. Ideally, good hygiene skills should be learned before you go to college. Many grooming activities such as shaving cause sensory discomfort. The person should try different shavers until they find one they can tolerate. It is often more comfortable to use unscented, hypoallergenic deodorant and cosmetics.

Choice of College Major

One problem I have observed is that a person with autism gets through college and then is unable to get a job. It is important to major in a field that will make the person employable. Some good majors are industrial design (that's my field), architecture, graphic art, computer science, statistics, accounting, library science, and special education. For people going to a community college, take courses such as architectural drafting, computer programming, or commercial art. Get really good at your skill. People respect talent.

Transition from College to Work

Individuals with ASD should start working part-time in their chosen field before they leave college. A slow transition from college to employment will be easier. While still in college do career relevant work each summer, even if it has to be on a volunteer basis. During my college years I worked on my aunt's ranch, in a research lab, and at a summer program for children with autism. I am seeing too many talented people graduating from college who have never held a job of any kind. It was this lack of job experience that made it difficult for them to find employment after college. They had no experience in being in a work environment, having to do tasks that other people assign, working alongside other people and the social requirements of doing so, or organizing their time and their workload, etc.

Finding Mentors and Appropriate Colleges

Over the years many people have asked me, "How did you find the mentors who helped you?" Mentors did, indeed, play a pivotal role in helping me become the person and professional I am today. They can be valuable catalysts to helping the spectrum child or teen learn fundamental study and research skills that will propel them toward a future career.

Mentors are attracted to ability. Many people will become interested in mentoring a child if they are shown examples of what the child is capable of doing. Portfolios of artwork, math, or writing can entice a potential mentor. A mentor can sometimes be found in the most unlikely places. He or she could be a retired engineer you sing beside in the church choir or a colleague at work.

When I was an inferior student in high school, my science teacher, Mr. Carlock, saved me by getting me interested in science. Our relationship started quite unexpectedly. The other teachers asked Mr. Carlock to talk to me because I was doing kind of "crazy talk" about the meaning of life. He explained that many of the ideas the other teachers thought were crazy were similar to the thoughts of well-known philosophers. He gave me books written by David Hume and other philosophers to whet my appetite to learn. After grabbing my interest this way, his next step was to motivate me to change my poor performance in class. He did this by saying, "If you want to find out why your squeeze machine is relaxing, you will need to study to become a scientist." He then took me to a big library to learn how real scientists search for journal articles. I read article after article about sensory perception. The library skills he taught me transferred easily to finding information on the internet. This is a good example of using my fixations to motivate my interest in schoolwork.

Parents, teachers, and friends need to always be on the lookout for possible mentors. Many retired individuals would love to work with a high school kid. Several individuals on the autism spectrum have gone into successful technical careers after being mentored by a retired person. It does not matter if the mentor's skills are old. What a mentor does is get a student turned on to learning. There is a discipline to learning a skill such as graphic design or computer programming. Once the mentor gets the student turned on, a spectrum person will go to the bookstore or the internet and buy the manuals to learn the modern techniques. I have observed that most teenagers on the autism spectrum need the discipline of formal instruction to get started. This is especially true in learning good study habits, researching information, and other related executive functioning skills, such as time management, group project strategies, etc.

Finding the Right College

I often get asked about colleges for individuals on the spectrum. There's no easy, quick answer to this question. I went to a small school—Franklin Pierce College in New Hampshire. Mother talked to the dean and they were willing to work with me. There are lots of small two-year and four-year colleges. A small school was ideal for my freshman and sophomore year because it avoided the problem of becoming lost in huge classes. The best approach is to identify a few schools that "fit" the person's needs, and then look for specific people in an institution who are willing to help.

Recently I have been doing a lot of talks at both large and small colleges. One school had an extensive department for helping students with disabilities and another small school emphasized hands-on learning in ecology and sustainable agriculture. The type of learning environments that appeal to the autistic way of thinking are often available. However, you need to seek out specific professors or counselors at both the community colleges and the four-year schools to help your child get in. Send a professor a portfolio of the student's work. One girl with Asperger's got into a top-ranked school after she sent her poetry to an English professor. You need to look for the "back door"—a professor who likes a student's work can let the student in.

To find an appropriate college, start your search on the internet. I typed in "colleges in Ohio," "colleges in Oregon," and "colleges in Alabama." I was amazed at the huge numbers of colleges in each state. Every college has a webpage and sub-webpages for each department, which usually offer a list of faculty. When I went to the University of Illinois, I was interested in the work of a specific professor because I had been reading his journal articles. The next step was visiting the university and talking to two professors about my interests. They admitted me to the graduate program, even though my standardized test scores were poor, because they were intrigued by my research ideas.

Being recognized in the cattle industry for my ability to design systems that worked was an added plus. Think creatively and find a back door into the college that is a good match for your child. A strong portfolio or an interesting idea for a research project may be the key. It's never too soon to start; the time to click the mouse is now.

When an individual with Asperger's graduates and gets out into the world of employment, it is often much wiser not to fully disclose.

Reasonable Accommodation for Individuals on the Autism Spectrum

I received an email recently from a woman with autism who is successfully partway through a Ph.D. program. She was inspired by my story and decided to get over her "handicapped mentality" and not let autism stand in the way of success. I am becoming more and more concerned about young students who are using high functioning autism or Asperger's as an excuse not to be able to do certain things. My mother insisted on standards of behavior such as good table manners, patient turn-taking, and not being rude. It is never too late to start teaching the essential social skills whether a person is two, twelve, or twenty.

In my opinion, some of the accommodations students are asking for in college are ridiculous and promote the handicapped mentality. One student expected the counseling department at a large university to intervene and stop a student who was using his mobile phone to text message in a huge class filled with over 200 students. To solve this problem, all she had to do was change seats to get away from the clicking keys. No one had taught her how to look for a simple solution first.

I have been receiving increasing complaints from college professors about students who disrupt classes and attempt to carry on a dialogue with the professor. When I was in college, I had a rule that I could ask a maximum of two questions per class period. Mr. Carlock, my science teacher, explained that the reason for this rule is to provide other students an opportunity to ask their questions. The principle is the same as turn-taking during board games or card games.

However, there are reasonable accommodations that are essential for some ASD individuals in college. A student may need just one or most of these accommodations.

- Taking exams in a room without fluorescent lights. I had a dyslexic student who totally "spaced out" and could not think in a room with fluorescent lights.
- Some extra time on tests.
- A quiet place to study; some individuals may need a private dorm room.
- Tutoring in some subjects.
- A lighter course load and taking an extra year to finish the degree.

At my university, more and more students want to take their exams in a private room at the Counseling Center. This creates a big hassle for the professor because that test paper is now separated from all the others. As a professor, I really dislike this because I write all my test questions on the blackboard. I do this to prevent students from archiving my old exams and using them as study guides. The reasonable accommodation I provide for these students is to allow them to take their tests in our department conference room. It has windows and the LED lights that flicker can be turned off. Students need to be taught to ask for a specific accommodation that helps with a specific problem, rather than a blanket request such as taking all quizzes and exams at the Counseling Center.

I have also talked to several professionals who work in the field of getting people on the spectrum employed. They share my concerns. One professional told me that at one college, Asperger's students were given less homework. I was never given less homework. A better alternative would be to take a lighter course load and go to college for an extra year. This has worked well for many AS students.

When an individual with ASD graduates and gets out into the world of employment, it is often much wiser to not fully disclose. This is especially important for the really smart, nerdy Asperger's kids. I received an email from a talented professional who was successfully employed for several years. He lost his job after he told his employer he had been diagnosed with Asperger's. It was discrimination and it was totally wrong. He needed no specific accommodation and disclosure opened the door to blatant discrimination. Often it is better to ask for a specific accommodation instead, such as having an office cube near a window to avoid fluorescent lights. Other examples of problems and solutions include:

- Difficulty with remembering long strings of verbal instruction. Tell the boss you prefer emailed instructions.
- Difficulty multi-tasking. Try to avoid these jobs if possible, or explain, "I'm not good at multi-tasking." Show your boss all the things you are really good at when you are not forced to multi-task.
- Need clear work objectives. Learn to ask lots of questions. I learned this in my design business. In order to achieve specific design objectives, I questioned the client extensively about the cattle-handling tasks he had to do in the corral. However, I never asked a client how he wanted a project designed. That was my job.

I am concerned that some individuals with ASD are getting a "handi-capped mentality" and think ASD renders them incapable of doing and achieving certain things. Or they feel their ASD diagnosis is a way out of doing the hard work that is required in life. This attitude will certainly hold them back from personal and professional success. In essence, they feel "less than"—which is not true. They are different from but not less than others. Reasonable accommodations exist to help an individual through tough spots. They aren't an excuse not to apply yourself in earnest to the tasks we all encounter in creating a life and a place for ourselves in the world.

Get Out and Experience Life!

I am seeing too many kids and young adults on the spectrum who are not getting out and doing things. They have turned into recluses who do not want to come out of their rooms. I was absolutely not allowed to do this. I had horrible anxiety attacks, but I still had to participate in activities at both school and home.

When I went away to boarding school at age 14, Mr. Patey, the headmaster at Hampshire Country School, had really good instincts on when to back off and let me do my own thing and when to insist on participation. When I became interested in taking care of cleaning stalls in the horse barn, this was encouraged because I was learning work skills. I was even given insulated boots so my feet would not freeze in the winter.

Mr. Patey drew one important line in the sand. He did not let me become a recluse in my room. I had to attend all meals and classes. He also insisted that I be on time. Every Sunday I had to dress appropriately for chapel and was required to attend. When I got really anxious and did not want to attend the campus movie night, he made me the projectionist. I had to participate with the school community.

Good and Bad Accommodations

Accommodations such as a quiet environment for study and extra time on tests are really helpful. But it is important to avoid accommodations that will reinforce a victim mentality. An example of a bad accommodation: allowing a student to do a public speaking assignment over the Internet. When I did my first public speaking in graduate school, I panicked and walked out. After that, I learned to use good audiovisual aids to give me cues and to prevent me from freezing up. When I did my first cattle-handling talks, I brought lots of pictures that illustrated behavioral principles. Creating excellent slides compensated for my early weak public speaking skills.

I often get asked about homeschooling. For some kids, this is a good option, but there must be lots of opportunities for social interaction with other children. I was teased and bullied and had to leave a large, regular high school. For some teenagers, finishing high school online would be the right thing to do. If you choose this option, the teenager *must* have opportunities to interact with peers and adults through activities, volunteer work, and job experience. Teens must learn work skills and how to cooperate in a work environment.

Trying New Things

For individuals on the spectrum to develop, they need to be "stretched" to try new things. When I was 15, I was afraid to go to my aunt's ranch. I really didn't want to go! Mother gave me a choice of going for either a week or all summer. When I got out to the ranch, I loved it and chose to stay all summer. I would have never known how much I loved working on a ranch if I had not given this experience a chance.

Developing Independence

Another problem I am observing is too many kids on the high end of the spectrum who are being overprotected and coddled. They are not learning how to independently perform tasks such as shopping, ordering food in restaurants, and practicing decent hygiene. Parents and teachers can encourage independence by taking kids out into the community. At first, the child should be accompanied by an adult during shopping or going on the bus. After a few trips, the individual can do it by himself.

Weighing Likes and Dislikes

There are individuals with ASD who get good jobs and then quit because they "don't like it." I have seen people on the spectrum leave good jobs with sympathetic bosses because they did not want to work. A vital lesson one has to learn is that you sometimes have to do stuff you don't like. I like my work as an animal science professor, but there are some tasks that are not fun. A good job has more tasks you like than tasks you hate. A person on the spectrum needs to learn that if he has a job where he is treated decently, but does not like the work, he should stick with it long enough to get a good recommendation for the next job.

Encourage your child to try new things, go new places, and develop new skills. Provide a variety of life experiences for your child as he grows. Allow your child to stretch beyond his comfort zone and relish the adventure!

Can My Adolescent Drive a Car?

Many parents ask me about the ability of people on the autism spectrum to drive a car. I have been driving since I was eighteen. I learned on the dirt roads at my aunt's ranch. Every day for an entire summer, I drove her old pickup truck three miles to the mailbox and back, which added up to 200 miles of driving. The truck had a manual gear shift and it would stall unless the clutch was worked just right. Because of the difficult clutch, for the first few weeks my aunt operated the clutch and I sat beside her, learning to steer. After I learned steering, it took me several weeks to master the clutch. Aunt Ann made sure I had completely mastered steering, braking, and changing gears before she let me drive the truck on a paved road with traffic.

The main difference between a typical adolescent and a person with autism is that more time may be required to master the skills involved in driving a car, and these skills may need to be learned one piece at a time. For instance, I didn't drive on a freeway until I was completely comfortable with slower traffic. The several months of driving in the safe, dirt roads on the farm provided the extra time I needed to learn safely.

Studies have shown that young adults with ASD perform more poorly in a driving simulator. To help improve these poor skills, the first step I recommend is practice. Practice operating the car in a big, safe place, such as a deserted parking lot or an open field.

When a motor skill, such as driving, is being learned, all people have to consciously think about the parts involved, such as steering or operating the clutch. During this phase of motor learning, the brain's frontal cortex is very active. When a skill such as driving or steering becomes fully learned, the person no longer has to think about performing the sequential steps involved. Steering the car becomes automatic and conscious thinking about how to do it is no longer required. At this point, the frontal cortex and other higher cortical regions are no longer activated. The subcortical region takes over when a skill is fully learned and the skill is executed unconsciously. Brain imaging studies conducted by researchers at the University of Oxford clearly showed how the brain switches to lower-level systems when a complex visual and motor task is fully learned.

I would recommend that the process of steering, braking, and otherwise operating a car be fully learned to the "motor automatic" stage before permitting your son or daughter to drive in any amount of traffic, or on a freeway. This helps solve the multi-tasking requirements involved with driving and frees up the frontal cortex to concentrate on traffic, rather than the operation of the car itself. When the individual first starts learning to drive, find some really safe places to practice, such as empty parking lots, open fields, or small country roads. One family had their child practice at an old closed military base.

If a child can ride a bike safely, and reliably obey the traffic rules, he or she can probably drive a car. When I was ten years old, I rode my bike everywhere and always obeyed the rules.

Likewise, to be able to drive a car, a person must already know how to steer a bike, golf cart, trike, electric wheelchair, or a toy vehicle. Parents interested in teaching their child to drive a car can plan ahead while the child is still young, making sure he or she first masters some of these skills on other types of vehicles. Do not get discouraged by students that show poor driving skills. Remember, baseline studies must be done BEFORE extensive driving practice is started. Performance will improve after lots of practice driving.

Another critical issue to consider is the maturity level of the individual. Does the boy or girl have enough mature judgment to drive a car? Are they careful to obey rules given them? How do they react under pressure? These factors need to be assessed on a case-by-case basis to determine if an adolescent is ready to tackle driving a car. I recommend allowing the person on the spectrum extra time to learn the basic operation of the car and the individual skills involved in driving. After each driving skill becomes fully learned and integrated with the other skills, they can slowly progress to driving on roads with more and more traffic, higher speeds, more frequent stops, or areas where there is a greater chance for different events to occur (for instance, driving in neighborhoods with lots of children or a high concentration of business establishments with cars pulling in and out of parking spaces regularly). Finally, nighttime driving should be avoided until the adolescent is very comfortable with all aspects of daytime driving.

I think rather than pondering, "Can my child with ASD drive a car," the more appropriate question is, "Is my child ready to drive a car?" The act of driving a car can be broken down into small, manageable pieces for instruction. The motor skills can be taught and, with enough practice, can be learned. However, driving is a serious matter, one that involves more than just learned skills. Each parent needs to decide whether or not their son or daughter has the maturity and good judgment required to allow them to get behind the wheel of a car. In this regard, the parents' decision is no different for a person on the spectrum than it would be for a typical child.

A new study shows that ASD individuals who learn to drive have safety records similar to normal drivers. Driver's Educational programs often put the individual with ASD onto roads with traffic too quickly. I recommend using one tank of gas and practice driving in a totally safe place, such as back roads, empty parking lots, or open fields. This will give the individual time to learn to operate the car before taking driver's education.

Additional Reading

Classen, S., Monahan, M., Hernandez, S. 2013. Indications of simulated driving skills in adolescents with autism spectrum disorder. *The Open Journal of Occupational Therapy* 1(4):2.

Curry, A. 2015. Driver licensing trajectories and motor vehicle crash rates among adolescents with autism spectrum disorders. American Public Health Association, online program 330458

Floyer, L.A. and Matthews, P.M. 2004. Changing brain networks for vaso-motor control with increased movement automaticity. *Journal of Neuropsychology* 92:2405-2412.

Reimer, R., et al. 2013. Brief report: examining driving behavior in young adults with high functioning autism spectrum disorders: a pilot study using a driving simulation paradigm. *Journal of Autism and Developmental Disorders* 43:2211-2217.

Through reading these articles, people with Asperger's also learn that even "normal" people have problems at work that cause stress and must be resolved.

Innovative Thinking Paves the Way for AS Career Success

Thorkil Sonne, the father of a child with Asperger's syndrome (AS), has founded a business in Denmark called Specialisterne Corporation that employs AS individuals to test new computer programs. Their job is to debug new software and their clients include Cryptomathic, a company that verifies digital signatures, and Case TDC, a major European telephone company. Testing new software is an ideal job for people with AS because the qualities of a good tester are some of the inherent strengths of a person with AS. Aspies have great memories, pay attention to details, are persistent, focused, and love structure.

Thorkil has created an innovative environment that is a win-win solution for both the employees and the corporation's clients. Because all the production employees have some degree of AS, on-the-job stress is reduced dramatically at Specialisterne Corporation. To further avoid daily stress and anxiety, work schedules are planned in advance. All tasks have well-defined goals and they are agreed upon in advance. Specialisterne will hire and train qualified AS job applicants. He uses the Lego Mindstorms programmable robots as a testing tool. That way, job applicants can demonstrate their programming skills with the robots instead of going through a formal interview process.

There are two things that Specialisterne does not tolerate: 1) anger where equipment is damaged or other people are hit, and 2) an individual who constantly stirs up gossip and conflict between coworkers. In return, the Aspies are provided with a work environment where sensory distractions are minimized and they do not have to deal with difficult bosses and complex social situations.

Today Specialisterne has three European offices and employs 50+ individuals, three quarters of whom are on the autism spectrum, to work with corporate clients. Major software companies such as SAP are now actively seeking people with autism because they have skills that are superior for debugging software.

AS-IT in Lincolnshire, England is another organization working with individuals with AS and high-functioning autism, in this case to train them for information technology positions in large corporations. Because of the "coaching" structure of AS-IT, it helps prevent problems with bosses who do not understand the AS employee. When a corporation hires one of AS-IT's trainees, he or she will still be able to stay in contact with AS-IT for assistance in the job transition as needed. Since the corporation knows they will be getting an AS employee, that, coupled with the increased awareness about autism and AS that AS-IT brings to the corporation, helps prevent misunderstandings when social situations develop that might have previously resulted in an AS individual being fired.

Over the years I have observed that the two main reasons a successful long-term Aspie employee was fired was because of 1) a new, unsympathetic boss and 2) the AS employee was promoted into a job that involved complex social skills and social interaction. The person may have been outstanding in a technical position such as a draftsman or engineer or programmer and he or she failed when promoted into a management position.

Employers need to be informed that promotion into management is not the best career path for AS individuals and many technical-type people.

These two corporations are using innovative thinking to design work environments in which people with AS can flourish.

The individuals with AS find the support they need in order to be successful and the corporations find brilliant minds that can propel their business forward. Win-win solutions like this are possible when neurotypicals start thinking outside the box and value the positive contributions that AS individuals have to offer.

Another approach to getting people with ASD employed is to create a company composed of people with ASD, but they do not advertise that they have ASD. I visited a successful animation company that used this approach. They found a niche business, which the big animation companies had been farming out to other countries. Now, instead of sending animation work such as movie titles and screen shading to India, clients are hiring these folks in the United States.

Another wide-open area is the skilled trades. Today, there is a huge shortage of automotive mechanics, machinists, plumbers, electrical utility workers, certified welders for the oil industry, and many others. Skilled trades are fields that will appeal to many visual and mathematical thinkers, and these jobs will never be outsourced to another country.

Resource

Wang, S. 2014. How autism can help you land a job. *Wall Street* Business Section, March 27, 2014.

Try on Careers

For all students, it is important to find a career that they are going to like. I get asked all the time – How did you get interested in the cattle industry? I came from a non-agricultural background and I became interested in the cattle industry when I visited my aunt's ranch at age 15. Students get interested in things they get exposed to. A big problem for many students on the autism spectrum is that they do not get exposed to enough new things. When a student is in both high school and college, they need to get employment in real jobs outside the home. The first job in high school teaches job skills and internships during college or apprenticeships let a student explore different careers.

Parents are often reluctant to get their child with autism out into the world. They are afraid that the child may become too anxious. When a teenager with autism finally gets out doing a job, they often blossom and love it. Some jobs where teens with autism have excelled are, an office supply store, bagging groceries, or an ice cream shop. In these jobs, the pace is slower and the teen can learn how to interact with customers. Since multi-tasking is often difficult a super busy fast food restaurant may be too hard. A busy store during the holiday season would be another poor choice. A common mistake made by parents teachers, or vocational counselors is, they do not differentiate between an individual where bagging groceries is a temporary training job and a more intellectually challenged person where it is an appropriate career. Research has shown that students on the spectrum who successfully keep jobs before they graduate, are often more successful in the work place. Getting and keeping jobs before graduation provides a gradual transition from the academic world to successful employment.

Opportunities for Individuals with ASD in the Skilled Trades

Today there is a big shortage of people in the high end skilled trades such as electricians, plumbers, welders who can build things from blueprints, mechanics, and heat and air conditioning technicians. These are good careers that will never get replaced by computers. I spent most of my career working with talented skilled trades people who built the livestock facilities that I designed. Many of these talented people were dyslexic or socially awkward. If these individuals had been children today, they would be in the special education department with an autism diagnosis. The people I worked with are now either retiring or getting ready to retire. They are not getting replaced. Due to the lack of new people entering the skilled trades, the U.S. is losing the skills to build industrial equipment. Equipment that is essential for industries, such as meat automated warehouses and food packaging, now have to be imported at great expense. We do not make it anymore. There are many individuals who might love a skilled trade. They will not know until they try it.

Introduce Students to Tools

The problem is that kids are growing up and they are not using tools. I have observed talented 16-year-olds who are still building with Legos because tools were never introduced. Removing hands-on skilled trades classes from the schools was a huge mistake. There are a few progressive school districts who are putting these classes back in. My kind of mind, the visual thinker, are often a perfect fit for skilled trades. There are kids who can build anything, but they cannot do algebra. Algebra is not needed for skilled trades. It must be removed as a barrier to the trades. A person who is really good at a highly skilled trade can have a job they will love for the rest of their career. The pay is good and there are full health benefits.

College Students on Spectrum Should do Summer Internships When They are in College

Each summer when a student is in college, they should do a different internship. This will enable them to try on careers and find out what they like. It is also equally important to find out what they hate. In the Animal Science Department at Colorado State University, we have many undergraduates who came from a non-agricultural background. They often get recruited to assist with research projects out in the beef industry. When these non-agricultural students experience working on a research project in either a large feedlot or meat plant; we discover that two usually love it and one hates it. A student will not find out what they will love or hate until they try it.

Today all students are encouraged to do internships when they are in college. Typical internships are designed to teach students how to solve problems and enable them to get to know a possible future employer. Interns no longer do menial work or just observe. They are usually assigned a real problem that they have to solve. Some examples of actual problems they had to solve during meat industry internships were: why was the automated warehouse losing boxes of meat? Or, what is the optimal speed to run a chicken wing processing line to get both efficiency and quality? An engineering student had to figure out why the electric forklifts were frequently running out of battery charge. After calling the company that made the forklifts, he learned that they were using the wrong charger. Students who can jump right in and solve these real problems will get hired.

The student also has to observe and learn how to work with other people to solve the problem. Some of these problems required an entire summer to solve. Not all internships involve factories. There are also internships at banks, insurance companies, and hospitals.

High school students with ASD who did project search job internships, 73% employed after high school. Controls with no internships only 17% employed after high school.

Further Reading

Gross, A. and Marus, J. (2018) High paying trade jobs sit empty, while high school graduates line up for university, *All Things Considered*, National Public Radio.

Adler, A.L. (2018) Chronic shortage of service techs threatens dealership profits, *Automotive News*, August 20, 2018.

Vopini, M. (2018) People with autism can help fill U.S. shortage of stem workers, *Dallas News*, February 7, 2018.

Wehman, P. et al. (2019) Competitive employment for transition age youth with significant impact with autism: A multi-site randomized clinical trial, *Journal of Autism and Developmental Disorders.*

The way I see it, it is likely that the genetics that produce autism are the same genetics that create an Einstein or a Mozart—it is more a matter of degree.

The Link Between Autism Genetics and Genius

A s a society, we still tend to view disabilities in a negative light. We may use politically correct language and say these people are "challenged" or "differently-abled," but the fact remains that we generally focus more on what they can't do, and tend to overlook the positive traits many of these individuals possess. Such is the case with people with autism and Asperger's Syndrome. If the genetic factors that cause autism were eliminated from the human race, we would pay a terrible price. The way I see it, it is likely that the genetics that produce autism are the same genetics that create an Einstein or a Mozart—it is more a matter of degree. A little of the genetic expression produces highly creative, brilliant thinkers. Too much of the genetics, however, results in severe autism, a nonverbal and much more challenged child.

If Albert Einstein were born today, he would be diagnosed with autism. He had no speech until age three, obsessively repeated certain sentences until the age of seven, and spent hours building houses from playing cards. His social skills remained odd through most of his life, and he was a self-described loner:

My passionate sense of social justice and social responsibility has always contrasted oddly with my pronounced lack of need for direct contact with other human beings and human communities. I am truly a lone traveler and have never belonged to my country, my home, my friends, or even my immediate family, with my whole heart. ...

A host of other brilliant historic figures such as Isaac Newton, Thomas Jefferson, Socrates, Lewis Carroll, Glenn Gould, and Andy Warhol are now speculated to have been on the autism spectrum.

Several books have been written that profile famous scientists, musicians, and artists who were on the autism/Asperger's spectrum. In his 2007 release, *Genius Genes: How Asperger Talents Changed the World*, Professor of Psychiatry at Trinity College, Dublin, Michael Fitzgerald, reached the conclusion that ASDs, creativity, and genius were all caused by similar genes, after comparing the characteristics of more than 1,600 people he had diagnosed with known biographical details of famous people. I see it the same way: A mild case of Asperger's Syndrome and being eccentric are the SAME thing, and the positive characteristics of being on the autism spectrum—detailed thinking, unwavering focus, obsessive interests in certain topics—are the very qualities that result in genius thought and world-changing discoveries. Simon-Baron Cohen, a researcher at the University of Cambridge, England, found that within families of children with autism, there existed a significantly greater number of parents and/or close relatives working as engineers and in other technical professionals. In my family, my grandfather was an MIT-trained engineer who was coinventor of the automatic pilot for airplanes.

Geeks, nerds, and eccentrics have always been in the world; what has changed is the world itself and our expectations of others within it. I work in a technical field and have worked with many engineers and other technical people who definitely displayed marked characteristics of Asperger's Syndrome. Most of these people are now in their forties, fifties, and sixties—and they are all undiagnosed. They were brought up in an era where social rules were more strictly defined and were carefully taught to all children. This more rigid upbringing actually helped these children acquire enough social skills to get by in the world.

Many are successful, and they have held good jobs for years. I know one Asperger's meat plant engineer who keeps a multimillion dollar plant running.

I get worried that today an Asperger's diagnosis may be detrimental to some individuals and hold them back. With greater competition for shrinking numbers of jobs, a person's social capabilities are now looked at as closely as are the person's technical skills or intellectual abilities. The most successful people with mild Asperger's work in places such as Silicon Valley, where superior talent still trumps social skills. Often these individuals have parents who are also in a high-tech field and as the child grew, placed more importance on teaching their children computer programming and other technical skills than worrying about whether or not they had girlfriends or boyfriends or wanted to attend every school dance.

I have given talks at conferences geared to a number of different diagnostic categories such as autism, gifted, and dyslexia. Even though diagnosis is not precise, each diagnostic group lives in its own world. When I go to the book tables, there are very few books stocked on *both* an autism book table and a gifted book table. The books addressing these individuals may be different but I see the same bright Asperger's kids at both autism and gifted children meetings. The Asperger's child at the gifted meeting is doing well in school, but the Asperger's child at an autism meeting may be in a poor special ed program, bored, and getting into trouble because adults in his life hold lower expectations of his abilities. Unfortunately, in some cases, people are so hung up on the labels attached to students that they teach to these low expectations and aren't even curious to learn if the child is actually more capable. This is mostly likely to occur when the label is Asperger's instead of gifted but developmentally delayed.

Parents and teachers should look at the child, not the child's label, and remember that the same genes that produce his Asperger's may have given the child the capacity to become one of the truly great minds of his generation. Be realistic with expectations, but don't overlook the potential for genius that may be quietly hiding inside, just waiting for an opportunity to express itself.

References

Baron-Cohen, S. 2000. Is Asperger syndrome/high functioning autism necessarily a disability? *Developmental Psychopathology* 12: 480-500.

Baron-Cohen, S., et al. 2007. Mathematical talent is linked to autism. *Human Nature* 18:125-131.

Einstein, A. 1954. *The World As I See It. In Ideas and Opinions, Based on Mein Weltbild*. Carl Seelig, editor. New York: Bonzana Books, pp. 8-11.

Fitzgerald, M., and B. O'Brien. 2007. *Genius Genes: How Asperger Talents Changed the World*. Shawnee Mission, KS: Autism Asperger Publishing Company.

Grandin, T. 2006. *Thinking in Pictures* (Expanded Edition). New York: Vintage/Random House.

Ledgin, N. 2002. *Aspergers and Self-Esteem: Insight and Hope through Famous Role Models.* Arlington, TX: Future Horizons, Inc. (This book profiles famous scientists and musicians who were probably Asperger's.)

Lyons, V., and Fitzgerald, M. 2013. Critical evaluation of the concept of autistic creativity. Intech. http://dx.doi. org/5772/54465

Soullieves, I. 2011. Enhanced mental image mapping in autism. *Neuropsychologia* 49:848-857.

Stevenson, J.L., and Gernsbacher, M.A. 2013. Abstract spatial reasoning on autistic strength. PLOS One. DOI: 10 1371/ journal. pone.0059329 .

My Sense of Self-Identity

O ne of my big concerns today is that too many children and teenagers on the autism spectrum are identifying so much with autism that it is hindering their pathway to success. When I was a teenager, I was fixated on science, horses, and the projects I built. These fixations were the basis of my self-identity and they helped propel me into a successful career. Today I am seeing smart individuals who have become so fixated on "their autism" that their entire lives revolve around it. When I was young, I talked endlessly about my favorite activities instead of autism. My fixations motivated me to create projects such as gates, horse bridles, carpentry work, and signs, which were all things other people wanted and appreciated. While creating these projects, I was also doing activities with other people. Teachers and parents need to work with both children and adults to get them involved in activities where they can have shared interests with other people, such as choir, art, auto mechanics, karate, working with animals, robot club, or drama club.

I have given several talks at large technical and computer conferences. At these conferences, I see lots of undiagnosed adults on the autism spectrum who have successful, high-level careers. All they talk about is the latest computer stuff; social chitchat bores them. Then the next day I travel to an autism conference and I meet a smart teenager who only wants to talk about autism. I would rather talk to him about an intense interest such as art, astronomy, history, or computers. It is fine to talk about autism, but it should not be the primary focus of an individual's life. Asperger's support groups are excellent because they enable individuals on the spectrum to communicate with others who have the same challenges. It is comforting for them to find out that they are not the only ones who are different.

However, there should be other activities so that the person's life does not totally center on autism. Parents are pivotal in making this happen in a child's life.

Several adults on the spectrum have talked to me about their autismcentric lives. They were either unemployed or had a boring, low-level job such as stocking shelves. I encouraged one of them to start a tutoring service and another to find activities involving music. They needed some activities that had nothing to do with autism. On the other hand, I have talked to older adults on the spectrum who have successful, high-level careers but in their personal lives, they felt empty. These individuals can really benefit from an autism/Asperger's support group.

At this stage in my adult life, being a college professor in the livestock industry is my primary identity and autism is secondary. Autism is an important part of me and I like my autistic logical way of thinking. I would never want to be cured and made "normal." To have a satisfying life, I do many things that have nothing to do with autism. The most successful people on the autism spectrum have either a career or activities they love to do. The nerds and the geeks at the computer conference were all kind of eccentric. Many were dressed in layered T-shirts like Sheldon wears in the television series *The Big Bang Theory*. Being eccentric is ok. I am kind of eccentric with my western clothes. In the HBO movie based on my life, there is a scene where a can of deodorant is slammed on the table and my boss says, "Use it, you stink." That actually happened, and today I thank my boss. It is fine to be eccentric but being dirty is not acceptable. There are too many teenagers and adults showing up in public unshaven or in messy clothes. I encourage people on the spectrum to be unique, but they should be neat. I met one man who taught college astronomy and he had a long ponytail and a cool astronomy T-shirt. I told him, "Don't let anybody tell you to cut your ponytail. Be a proud geek who can excel in an interesting career."

Now that I'm 72, looking back on my life, I remember how I spent a lot of time during my twenties trying to figure out the ultimate meaning of life. I suppose that is not very different from other young adults at that age, as we try to define ourselves and find our own way. Today I find meaning in doing things that make real, positive changes in the world. When a mother tells me that reading my book helped her understand her child, or when a rancher tells me that the corrals I designed work well, that provides meaning to my life.

Tony & Temple:
Face to Face

T emple Grandin's autobiography *Emergence: Labeled Autistic* and her subsequent book, *Thinking in Pictures,* together contain more information and insights into autism than I have read in any textbook. When I first heard one of her presentations, I was immediately aware of her forthright personality. The whole audience was enthralled with her knowledge.

I was delighted to be asked to interview Temple, as it provided an opportunity to seek her counsel on so many topics. She has a remarkably endearing personality and during the interview in San Francisco she entranced an audience of over 300 people. The applause at the end was loud and prolonged.

Temple is my hero. She has my vote for the person who has provided the greatest advance in our understanding of autism this century.

— Dr. Tony Attwood
World-renowned expert on autism
and Asperger's Syndrome

Ed. Note: The following interview was taped live on December 9, 1999 at a presentation Temple was giving in San Francisco for Future Horizons. The audience loved it! It provided many revealing, and sometimes humorous, glimpses into Temple's life. It was a rare opportunity to see Temple break into hearty laughter. Enjoy!

TONY: Temple, you were diagnosed as autistic when you were fifteen years old. How did your parents present that to you and what did you feel about yourself when you got that information?

TEMPLE: Well, they never really presented it properly. I sort of found out about it in a roundabout way from my aunt. You've got to remember that I'm a child of the '50s and that was a Freudian era, a totally different time. Actually, I was kind of relieved to find out there was something wrong with me. It explained why I wasn't getting along with the other kids at school and I didn't understand some of the things teenagers did—like when my roommate would swoon over the Beatles. She'd roll around on the floor squealing in front of *The Ed Sullivan Show*. I'd think, yeah, Ringo's cute, but I wouldn't roll around on the floor with him. ...

TONY: So, if you had the job of explaining to a fourteen or fifteen-year-old that you have autism or Asperger's Syndrome, how would you talk about it today?

TEMPLE: I think I might give them your book and my book. ... Well, I'd probably just explain it in a technical manner: that it's immature development in the brain that interferes with getting along socially. I'm basically a "techie"—that's the kind of person I am. I want to fix things. With most of the things I do, I take the engineering approach; my emotions are simple. I get satisfaction out of doing good work. I get satisfaction when a parent comes to me and says "I read your book and it really helped my kid in school." I get satisfaction from what I do.

TONY: I seem to remember when you were very little and very autistic, there were certain autistic behaviors you really enjoyed doing. What were they?

TEMPLE: One of the things I used to do was dribble sand through my hands and watch the sand, studying each little particle like a scientist looking at it under a microscope. When I did that I could tune the whole world out. You know, I think it's okay for an autistic kid to do a little bit of that, because it's calming. But if they do it all day, they're not going to develop. Lovaas' research showed that kids need forty hours a week connected to the world. I don't agree with forty hours a week of what I call "hard-core applied behavior analysis," just done at a table. But I had forty hours a week of being tuned in. I had an hour and-a-half a day of Miss Manners meals where I had to behave. Then nanny played structured children's games with me and my sister, ones that involved a lot of turn-taking. I had my speech therapy class every day ... these things were very important to my development.

TONY: A moment ago you used the word "calming." One of the problems that some persons with autism and Asperger's have is managing their temper. How do you control your temper?

TEMPLE: When I was a little kid, if I had a temper tantrum at school, mother just said, "You're not going to watch any Howdy Doody show tonight." I was in a normal school—twelve kids in a class, a structured classroom. There was a lot of coordination between school and home. I knew I couldn't play Mom against the teachers, or vice versa. I just knew if I had a temper tantrum there wouldn't be any TV that night. When I got into high school and kids were teasing me, I got into some rather serious fist fights. I got kicked out of the school for that—it was not good. And then when I went away to the boarding school and I got into some fist fights, they took away horseback riding privileges. Well, I wanted to ride the horses and after I had horseback-riding privileges taken away once, I stopped fighting. It was just that simple.

TONY: But can I ask you, personally, whom were you fighting, and did you win?

TEMPLE: Well ... I usually won a lot of the fights ...

TONY: So, were you fighting the boys or the girls?

TEMPLE: Both—the people who teased me.

TONY: So you'd actually lay out the boys?

TEMPLE: Oh, I remember one time I punched a boy right in the cafeteria ... and then when I stopped fighting, the way I dealt with it was that I would just cry, because it's my way of preventing fighting. I also avoid situations where people are blowing up and getting angry. I just walk away from them.

TONY: I'd like to ask you a technical question. If you had $10 million for research and you were either going to create research in new areas, or support existing research, where would you spend that money?

TEMPLE: One of the areas I would spend it on is really figuring out what causes all the sensory problems. I realize it's not the core deficit in autism, but it's something that makes it extremely difficult for persons with autism to function. Another really bad thing, especially in the high-functioning end of the spectrum, is that as the people get older, they get more and more anxious. Even if they take Prozac or something else, they're so anxious, they have a hard time functioning. I wish there was some way to control that without drugging them totally to death. Then you get into issues like, should we prevent autism? I get concerned about that because if we totally get rid of the genetics that cause autism, then we'd be getting rid of a lot of talented and gifted people, like Einstein. I think life is a continuum of normal to abnormal. After all, the really social people are not the people who make computers, who make power plants, who make big hotel buildings like this one. The social people are too busy socializing.

TONY: So, you wouldn't fund getting rid of Asperger's Syndrome. You don't see it as a tragedy?

TEMPLE: Well, it would be nice to get rid of the causation for the severely impaired, if there was a way we could preserve some of the genetics, too. But the problem is that there are a lot of different interacting genes. If you get a little bit of the trait, it's good; you get too much of the trait, it's bad. It seems to be how genetics works. One thing I've learned from working with animals, when breeders over select for a certain trait, you can get other bad things that come along with it. For example, with chickens, they are selected for fast growth and lots of meat, but then they had problems with the skeleton not being strong enough. So they bred a strong skeleton back into the chicken. And they got a big, rude surprise they weren't expecting.

They ended up with roosters that the breeding hens were attacking and slashing. When they bred the strong legs back in, it bred out the rooster's normal courtship behavior. Now, who would have predicted this strange problem? That's the way genetics works.

TONY: Temple, one characteristic you have is that you make people laugh. I think sometimes you may not intend it, but you have a great gift of making people laugh. What makes you laugh? What's your sense of humor?

TEMPLE: Well for one thing, my humor is visually based. When I was telling you about the chickens, I was seeing pictures of them. One time I was in our department conference room at the university. They have framed pictures of all the old department heads, in heavy, thick, wooden frames. I looked at that and said, "Oh, framed geezers!" At another faculty meeting I was looking at them, and I wanted to burst out laughing, thinking about the framed geezers. That's visual humor.

TONY: And you have a story about pigeons?

TEMPLE: Oh yeah, the pigeon stuff. Wayne and I got rolling around on the ground one night about pigeons. The Denver airport has a lot of pigeons and they don't clean up the dead pigeons in the parking lot. I got to thinking about the places I could put the dead pigeons ... like a pigeon hood-ornament for all the city of Denver maintenance trucks. Then they have this place they call the pigeon drop zone. In the parking garage there's this one concrete beam where they all nest ... well you don't want to park in the pigeon drop zone. Every time I walk back to the parking garage, I'm wondering what big fancy expensive $30,000 SUV just parked in the pigeon drop zone.

TONY: So, that explains why sometimes you may burst into laughter and other people have no idea what's going on. ...

TEMPLE: That's right; it's because I'm looking at a picture in my mind of something that's funny ... I can just see that pigeon hood-ornament on a bright yellow Denver city truck—it's just very funny.

TONY: About your family: your mother was a very important part of your life. What sort of a person is she? What did she do personally that helped you?

TEMPLE: She kept me out of an institution, first of all. You've got to remember this was fifty years ago; all of the professionals recommended that I be put into an institution. Mother took me to a really good neurologist and the neurologist recommended the speech therapy nursery school. That was just a piece of luck. The nursery school was run by two teachers out of their house. They had six kids and they weren't all autistic. They were just good teachers who knew how to work with kids. They hired the nanny, when I was three, and the nanny had had experience working with autistic kids. I have a feeling the nanny might have been Asperger's herself, because she had an old car seat out of a jeep that she had in her room—it was her favorite chair.

TONY: How else did your mother help you as a person herself?

TEMPLE: Well, she worked with me a lot. She encouraged my interest in art; she did some drawing things with me. She had worked as a journalist, putting together a TV show on mentally disabled persons and then another TV program on emotionally disturbed children. Of course, back then, fifty years ago, different children were all labeled as emotionally disturbed. As a journalist, she had gone out and visited different schools. So when I got into trouble in ninth grade for throwing a book at a girl—I got kicked out of the school and we had to find another school—she found a boarding school that was one of the schools she had visited as a journalist. If she hadn't done that for me, I don't know what would have happened. Once I got into the boarding school, that's when I found people like my science teacher and my Aunt Ann, out on the ranch, who were other important mentors. But there were a lot of people along the way who helped me.

TONY: What about your father? Describe your father and grandfather.

TEMPLE: My grandfather on my mother's side invented the automatic pilot for airplanes. He was very shy and quiet; he wasn't very social. On my father's side of the family we have temper problems. My father didn't think I would amount to very much. He wasn't very social either.

TONY: How do you relax? What do you do to calm down at the end of the day?

TEMPLE: Before I took medication I used to watch *Star Trek*—I was very much a Trekkie. One of the things I liked, especially about the old classic *Star Trek*, was that it always had good moral principles. I'm very concerned today about all the violent stuff. It isn't so much how many guns are going off in the movies, it's that the hero doesn't have good values. When I was a little kid, Superman and the Lone Ranger never did anything that was wrong. Today, we have heroes that do things like throw the woman into the water or the woman ends up getting shot; the hero is supposed to be protecting the woman, not letting her get shot. You don't have clear-cut values. And this worries me, because my morals are determined by logic. What would my logic and morals have become if I hadn't been watching those programs, with clear-cut moral principles?

TONY: As we turn to the next millennium, in another 100 years time, how do you think our understanding of autism will change?

TEMPLE: Oh, I don't know ... we'll probably have total genetic engineering and they'll have a Windows 3000 "Make a Person" program. They'll know how to read DNA code by then. We don't know how to do that right now. Scientists can manipulate DNA—take it out and put it in—but they cannot read the four-base source code. One hundred years from now they'll be able to do that. And, I don't think there will be autism, at least not the severe forms of it, because we'll be able to totally manipulate the DNA by then.

TONY: There are a number of persons we've learned about now with autism or Asperger's Syndrome who have written their autobiographies. Who are your heroes in the autism/Asperger's field who have the condition themselves?

TEMPLE: I really look to the people who have made a success of themselves. There's a lady named Sara Miller; she programs industrial computers for factory automation. There's a lady here tonight, very beautifully dressed, who has her own jewelry business, and she told me she has Asperger's. Somebody like that is my hero ... somebody who's making a success of himself or herself, who is getting out there and doing things.

TONY: How about famous people historically, who would you think had autism or Asperger's Syndrome?

TEMPLE: I think Einstein had a lot of autistic traits. He didn't talk until age three—I have a whole chapter about Einstein in my last book. I think Thomas Jefferson had some Asperger's traits. Bill Gates has tremendous memory. I remember reading in an article that he memorized the whole Torah as a child. It's a continuum—there's just no black and white dividing line between a computer techie and say, an Asperger's person. They just all blend right together. So if we get rid of the genetics that cause autism, there might be a horrible price to pay. Years ago, a scientist in Massachusetts said if you got rid of all the genes that caused disorders, you'd have only dried up bureaucrats left!

To conclude, Tony opened up the interview to questions from the audience. Here's one of the best.

AUDIENCE MEMBER: How did you realize you had control over your life?

TEMPLE: I was not a good student in high school; I did a lot of fooling around. Being a visual thinker, I had to use door symbolism—an actual physical door that I would practice walking through—to symbolize that I was going on to the next step in my life. When you think visually, and you don't have very much stuff on the [mental] hard drive from previous experiences, you've got to have something to use as a visual map. My science teacher got me motivated with different science projects and I realized if I wanted to go to college and become a scientist, I'd have to study. Well, one day I made myself walk through this one door and I said, "Okay, I'm going to try to study during French class." But there was a point where I realized that I had to do something about my own behavior. And I had experienced sometimes that were not all that easy, like when my boss got all over me for being a total slob. There were mentors who forced me—and it wasn't always pleasant—but they forced me to realize that I had to change my behavior. People on the spectrum just can't be sitting around complaining about things. They have to actively try to change things. Good mentors can help you do that.

Dr. Tony Attwood is a clinical psychologist from Brisbane, Australia, with over thirty years of experience with individuals with autism, Asperger's Syndrome, and Pervasive Developmental Disorder (PDD). He has worked with several thousand individuals, from infants to octogenarians, from profoundly disabled persons to university professors. His books and videos on Asperger's Syndrome and high-functioning autism are recognized as the best offerings in the field. Over 300,000 copies of his book *Asperger's Syndrome: A Guide for Parents and Professionals*, have been sold, and it has been translated into twenty languages.

Bibliography

Most articles appearing in this book are selections from an exclusive column written by Temple Grandin in the award-winning national magazine on ASD, the *Autism Asperger's Digest*. Find information about the *Digest* at www.autismdigest.com.

Chapter 1: The Importance of Early Education

Do Not Get Trapped by Labels. *May-June 2014*

Economical Quality Programs for Young Children with ASD. *September-October 2005*

Different Types of Thinking in Autism. *November-December 2005*

Higher Expectations Yield Results. *March-April 2007*

Teaching Turn Taking. *June-July 2014*

What School is Best for My Child with ASD? *April-May 2012*

Chapter 2: Teaching and Education

Finding a Child's Area of Strength. *September-October 2009*

Teaching How to Generalize. *November-December 2000*

The Importance of Developing Talent. *January-February 2001*

Teaching People with Autism/Asperger's to be More Flexible. *July-August 2002*

Teaching Concepts to Children with Autism. *November-December 2003*

Bottom-Up Thinking and Learning Rules. *September-October 2010*

Laying the Foundation for Reading Comprehension. *January-February 2014*

Motivating Students. *September-October 2004*

Getting Kids Turned On to Reading. *November-December 2007*

Managing Video Game Use. *July-August 2012*

Service Dogs and Autism. *March-April 2011*

The Importance of Choices. *November-December 2013*

The Importance of Practical Problem-Solving Skills. *March-April 2008*

Learning to do Assignments Other People will Appreciate. *November-December 2008*

Learning Never Stops. *November-December 2009*

Service Dogs and Autism. *March-April 2011*

Chapter 3: Sensory Issues

Visual Processing Problems in Autism. *July-August 2004*

Auditory Problems in Autism. *November-December 2004*

Incorporating Sensory Integration into your Autism Program. *March-April 2005*

The Effect of Sensory and Perceptual Difficulties on Learning Styles. *November-December 2006*

Environmental Enrichment Therapy for Autism. *November-December 2014*

Chapter 4: Understanding Nonverbal Autism

A Social Teenager Trapped Inside. *September-October 2012*

You Asked Me! *January-February 2002*

Why Do Kids with Autism Stim? *September-October 2011*

Tito Lives in a World of Sensory Scrambling. *May-June 2005*

Understanding the Mind of a Nonverbal Person with Autism. *March-April 2009*

Solving Behavior Problems in Nonverbal Individuals with Autism. *May-June 2005*

Whole-Task Teaching for Individuals with Severe Autism. *September-October 2007*

Chapter 5: Behavior Issues

Disability versus Just Bad Behaviors. *May-June 2003*

Innovative Methods for Handling Hitting, Biting, and Kicking. *January-February 2009*

My Experience with Teasing and Bullying. *July-August 2001*

Rudeness is Inexcusable. *May-June 2006*

The Need to Be Perfect. *January-February 2010*

Autism and Religion: Teach Goodness. *May-June 2002*

Chapter 6: Social Functioning

Insights into Autistic Social Problems. *November-December 2002*

Learning Social Rules. *January-February 2005*

Emotional Differences among Individuals with Autism or Asperger's. *September-October 2006*

Healthy Self-Esteem. *May-June 2007*

Four Cornerstones of Social Awareness. *July-August 2007*

Questions about Connecticut Shooter Adam Lanza, Asperger's Syndrome, and SPD. *Sensory Focus Magazine, Spring 2013*

Chapter 7: Medications & Biomedical Therapy

Alternative versus Conventional Medications. *March-April 2004*

Hidden Medical Problems Can Cause Behavior Problems. *May-June 2009*

Evaluating Treatments. *May-June 2004*

Medication Usage: Risk versus Benefit Decisions. *July-August 2005*

My Treatment for Ringing in the Ears. *March-April 2010*

Chapter 8. Cognition and Brain Research

Brain Cortex Structure Similar in Brilliant Scientists and Autism. *January-February 2008*

A Look Inside the Visual-Thinking Brain. *January-February 2007*

The Role of Genetics and Environmental Factors in Causing Autism. *July-August 2009*

Chapter 9: Adult Issues and Employment

Improving Time Management and Organizational Skills. *January-February 2012*

Employment Advice: Tips for Getting and Holding a Job. *May-June 2001*

Teens with ASD Must Learn Both Social and Work Skills to Keep Jobs. *September-October 2013*

Happy People on the Autism Spectrum have Satisfying Jobs or Hobbies. *March-April 2002*

Inside or Outside? The Autism/Asperger's Culture. *November-December 2001*

Portfolios Can Open Job and College Opportunities. *May-June 2013*

Going to College: Tips for People with Autism & Asperger's. *March-April 2001*

Finding Mentors and Appropriate Colleges. *July-August 2010*

Reasonable Accommodation for Individuals on the Autism Spectrum. *May-June 2010*

Get Out and Experience Life! *July-August 2013*

Can My Adolescent Drive a Car? *March-April 2003*

Innovative Thinking Paves the Way for AS Career Success. *March-April 2006*

The Link Between Autism Genetics and Genius. *July-August 2008*

My Sense of Self-Identity. *November-December 2010*

About the Author

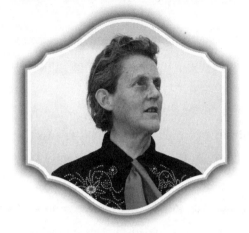

T emple Grandin, PhD, didn't talk until she was 3½ years old, communicating her frustration instead by screaming, peeping, and humming. In 1950, she was diagnosed with autism, and her parents were told she should be institutionalized. She tells her story of "groping her way from the far side of darkness" in her book *Emergence: Labeled Autistic*, a book that stunned the world because, until its publication, most professionals and parents assumed that an autism diagnosis was virtually a death sentence to achievement or productivity in life.

Dr. Grandin has become a prominent author and speaker on the subject of autism because:

> I have read enough to know that there are still many parents, and yes, professionals too, who believe that 'once autistic, always autistic.' This dictum has meant sad and sorry lives for many children diagnosed, as I was in early life, as autistic. To these people, it is incomprehensible that the characteristics of autism can be modified and controlled. However, I feel strongly that I am living proof that they can.
>
> —Temple Grandin in *Emergence: Labeled Autistic*

Even though she was considered "weird" in her young school years, she eventually found a mentor who recognized her interests and abilities. Dr. Grandin later developed her talents into a successful career as a livestock-handling equipment designer, one of very few in the world. She has now designed the facilities in which half of the cattle in the United States are handled, and she consults for firms such as Burger King, McDonald's, and Swift.

Dr. Grandin is now the most accomplished and well-known adult with autism in the world. Her fascinating life, with all its challenges and successes, has been brought to the screen. She has been featured on National Public Radio and major television programs, such as the BBC special "The Woman Who Thinks Like a Cow," ABC's *Primetime Live*, *The Today Show*, *Larry King Live*, *48 Hours*, and *20/20*, and has been written about in many national publications, such as *Time* magazine, *People* magazine, *Forbes*, *U.S. News and World Report*, and *The New York Times*. Among numerous other recognitions in the media, Bravo aired a program about her life, and she was featured in the best-selling book, *Anthropologist from Mars*.

Dr. Grandin presently works as a Professor of Animal Science at Colorado State University. She also speaks around the world on both autism and cattle handling.

Dr. Grandin's current best-selling book on autism is *The Way I See It: A Personal Look at Autism*. She also authored *Unwritten Rules of Social Relationships*, *Animals Make Us Human*, *Animals in Translation*, *Thinking in Pictures*, and *Emergence: Labeled Autistic* and produced several DVDs.